OXFORD MEDICAL PUBLICATIONS

The Principles of Endodontics

DATE DUE

The Principles of Endodontics

Michael Manogue BDS, MDSc, PhD, FDS, MRD, DRD RCS (Ed)

Director of Learning and Teaching
Leeds Dental Institute
UK

Shanon Patel BDS, MSc, MClinDent, MFDS RCS (Eng), MRD RCS (Ed)

Postgraduate Endodontic Unit
King's College London
UK

Richard T. Walker RD, BDS, PhD, MSc, FDS RCS (Eng), FDS RCPS (Glasg)

Former Centre Director
International Centre for Excellence in Dentistry
Eastman Dental Institute for Oral Health Sciences
University College London
UK

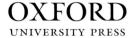

OXFORD
UNIVERSITY PRESS

OXFORD
UNIVERSITY PRESS

Great Clarendon Street, Oxford OX2 6DP

Oxford University Press is a department of the University of Oxford.
It furthers the University's objective of excellence in research, scholarship,
and education by publishing worldwide in

Oxford New York

Auckland Cape Town Dar es Salaam Hong Kong Karachi Kuala Lumpur Madrid
Melbourne Mexico City Nairobi New Delhi Taipei Toronto Shanghai

With offices in

Argentina Austria Brazil Chile Czech Republic France Greece Guatemala Hungary
Italy Japan South Korea Poland Portugal Singapore Switzerland Thailand Turkey
Ukraine Vietnam

Oxford is a registered trade mark of Oxford University Press
in the UK and in certain other countries

Published in the United States
by Oxford University Press Inc., New York

A catalogue record for this title is available from the British Library

Data available

Library of Congress Cataloguing in Publication Data

Manogue, Michael.
The Principles of Endodontics / Michael Manogue, Shanon Patel, Richard T. Walker.
Includes bibliographical references and index.
1. Endodontics. [DNLM: 1. Endodontics–methods.   WU 230 M285p 2005]   I. Patel,
Shanon.   II. Walker, R. T.   III. Title. RK351.MS66 2005   617.6'342–dc22
2005006670

ISBN 0 19 8509995 (Pbk)   978 0 19 850 999 8

10 9 8 7 6 5 4 3 2 1

Typeset by EXPO Holdings Sdn Bhd., Malaysia
Printed in Great Britain
on acid-free paper by Ashford Colour Press Limited, Gosport, Hampshire

We would like to acknowledge the inspiration provided by dental students, past and present and the unfailing support of our families, particularly Kate, Maggie, and Almas, in the preparation of this book.

Foreword

To demystify endodontics, for the undergraduate dental student in particular, is the very worthwhile aim of this textbook.

Without a clear understanding of the 'Why' of endodontics, no student can hope to achieve a consistently high standard in their clinical practice. The authors do address the 'Why?' and then the 'How?' by dividing the text into two main sections, each being similarly subdivided into pertinent topics. The result is not only easy to read and comprehend, but the colour coding makes both aspects of each topic easy to locate, an important factor in holding the attention and interest of the reader.

The informal style and lightness of touch will not intimidate the novice endodontist but will go a long way to imparting the basic understanding so necessary for clinical success. The authors are very obviously crusaders in their quest for higher standards in endodontics and where better to start than with the undergraduate student or those wishing to refresh their knowledge? With this in mind, the third and most challenging section of the text is dedicated to self-assessment by the reader, thus encouraging evaluation of their understanding through careful consideration of specific clinical cases relevant to each chapter.

By using the understanding and self awareness so clearly imparted here, enthusiasm for endodontics will be enkindled at an early stage and result in keenness to undertake clinical practice to the highest standards in what is a most exacting part of dentistry.

Dr Elizabeth M Saunders
Dundee
January 2005

Preface

This book provides a simple approach to the principles of endodontics. It has been written, principally, for the dental student who is new to the discipline and repeated references are made to 'you' the student and variations in practice that may occur in 'your' dental school. This is not to say that there may be nothing here for the more experienced student or recent graduate, because an alternative approach sometimes provides an opportunity to re-enthuse or the explanation of a concept in another way may allow clearer formulation of thought. Indeed, there is scope here for the potential candidate preparing for the IQE and background information for those studying for MFDS. The fundamental principle of the text is 'Why?'—many of us can produce a satisfactory technical result, but not everyone may understand the reasons, for example, of the progression of disease or what determines success or failure of treatment.

The authors have a very broad range of experience in clinical dentistry and dental education; their differing backgrounds and experience (from specialist practitioner to academic) has made for stimulating discussion in the preparation of the text and, hopefully, the development of an accessible and educational book.

The book is arranged in three distinct, but related, sections and is colour coded to encourage the reader to move between areas of interest. Section A covers the theory of endodontology (the 'Why?' section), moving from the life of a tooth from development to demise, through preservation of pulp vitality to the principles of preparation and obturation and concludes with evaluation of the outcome of root canal treatment and management of failure. Section B comprises a shorter, very practical guide (the 'How?' section) to the practice of endodontics. It has several lists of criteria for determining success in the various aspects of endodontic treatment. This is an attempt to articulate the bare minimum required and in so doing may be somewhat contentious. Section C poses a series of self-assessment questions about clinical cases focused on the preceding chapters. It also provides answers—but the reader is encouraged to ask themselves whether they are able to answer them first!

Throughout, there are instances where the reader will be invited to stop and think about what they are doing and their approach to the discipline. In Section B, for example, there are specific examples of where self-assessment might be found useful. The authors are particularly interested in endorsing the theory that it is through the process of developing accuracy of criterion-based self-assessment and reflection that encouragement will be found to lead to improvement in clinical practice. Self-assessment has been described as the key to lifelong learning and annoying as it may at first appear, we urge you to think critically as you read. If you, or your tutors, disagree with what is stated in the book, surely that must be better than merely accepting everything that is placed before you. Through that irritation will come formulation of concepts and goals that are your own.

We make no pretences and it may be that the simple style adopted will not be to everyone's taste, but it seemed plain to us that there was space in the literature for a very practical guide to this fascinating, frustrating, hugely worthwhile aspect of clinical dentistry. We wish you success, enjoyment and *understanding* in your clinical practice.

Michael Manogue, Leeds
Shanon Patel, London
Dick Walker, Ilkley
February 2005

Acknowledgements

The authors would like to acknowledge the help of the following in the preparation of this book:

Especial thanks go to Maria Lessani, for her significant contributions to the early drafts, and to Kishor Gulabivala whose input was invaluable.

A few images were kindly supplied by our colleagues. These are indicated in the text.

We would also like to thank the staff at OUP, in particular Catherine Barnes, Commissioning Editor, for unstinting support, patience, and advice.

Contents

Section A

Theory

Introduction

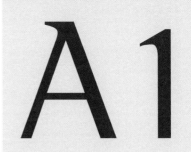

Introduction

Why endodontics?

The term 'endodontics' literally means within teeth. The practical aspects of the subject can only be mastered and developed when the scientific foundations of the discipline are clearly comprehended.

Definitions

The teeth and their supporting tissues may become involved in dental infections that are caused by microorganisms from the oral flora. These microorganisms have their effects either around (prefix—*perio*) or within (prefix—*endo*) teeth.

Periodontal diseases affect the periodontal attachment apparatus and the tissues around the tooth (Fig. A1.1). This results in loss of bony support for the teeth.

Periodontology is the branch of dental science that deals with the form of, function of, health of, and diseases affecting the periodontal tissues.

Periodontics is described as the clinical discipline that is involved with the prevention, diagnosis, and treatment of periodontal disease.

A similar approach may be adopted when describing endodontic biology. Infections occurring within teeth may be termed *endodontal diseases*. They are usually characterized by loss of integrity of the crown, invasion by microorganisms, and destruction of enamel, dentine, and ultimately, the dental pulp. Dental caries provides a good example of an endodontal disease. There is dissolution of the enamel, invasion of the dentinal tubules, demineralization and destruction of the dentine, and eventual pulpal involvement (Fig. A1.2). Trauma, tooth surface loss, and microleakage around restorations may also lead to endodontal infection.

Endodontology may be defined as the branch of dental science concerned with the form, function, health, injuries to and diseases of the dentine and dental pulp.

Endodontics is the clinical discipline that deals with the prevention, diagnosis, and treatment of endodontal (endodontic) disease. In essence, this involves all procedures required for the maintenance of the health of vital teeth and, where teeth have become infected, procedures designed to eradicate the effects of microorganisms and retain teeth as functional units in the dental arch.

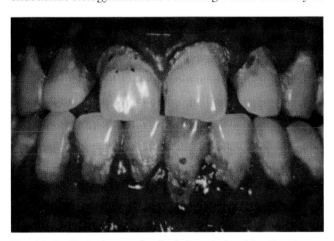

Fig. A1.1 Clinical example of adult periodontitis. Courtesy of Dr G. Auplish

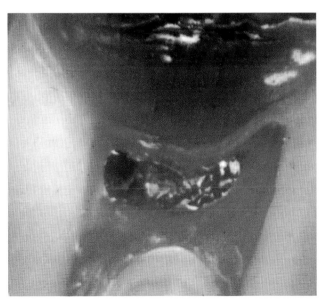

Fig. A1.2 Section of tooth with caries, dentine destruction, and pulp involvement.

Basis for clinical practice

Understanding endodontics requires knowledge of the biological processes affecting the oral tissues and other related basic science subjects that support this understanding. They include:

- the embryology of the oral tissues with particular reference to the formation of the dental tissues of the teeth and jaws;
- the gross and surgical anatomy of the head and neck;
- the histology of the oral tissues including the composition and structure of enamel and dentine;
- the physiology of the dental tissues emphasizing the role of pulp and the periradicular tissues;
- the pathological processes that might affect the head and neck;
- the specific processes involved in the diseases of the pulp and periradicular tissues;
- oral microbiology and the clinical relevance of the oral microflora with a detailed knowledge of the ways in which dental infection develops;
- the pharmacological benefits of the drugs used in general dentistry and endodontics;
- the science of the instruments and materials used in endodontic practice.

Which clinical conditions require management?

Patients requiring endodontic treatment generally present with and complain about oro-facial pain, swelling, or both. However, endodontal disease affecting the pulp and periradicular tissues may also occur in the absence of pain or swelling.

The clinician, using his/her in-depth knowledge of the biology and pathology of the oral tissues, should be able to listen to and communicate with the patient and, with the aid of diagnostic tests, arrive at a diagnosis. On the basis of this diagnosis, following an analysis of patient acceptance and expectations and the operator's own level of competence, treatment is prescribed and provided within a framework of the total oral care needs of the patient.

The clinical conditions that are likely to require endodontic treatment are:

- dental caries;
- painful and non-painful pulpitis;
- painful and non-painful periradicular periodontitis;
- suppurative periradicular periodontitis (chronic abscess);
- acute periradicular abscess;
- traumatized and cracked teeth;
- internal and external root resorption.

What are the scope and aims of treatment?

Endodontics has come of age and now occupies an important position in the general dental care of patients. No longer is the subject synonymous with only root canals and root canal treatment. It has taken on a much wider responsibility in the area of dental diseases and the treatment of infections involving the teeth. The science and art of this clinical discipline encompasses:

- diagnosis of oro-facial pain;
- preservation of healthy dental pulps;
- root canal treatment involving pulp space disinfection and sealing;
- traumatology;
- surgical endodontics.

Where endodontic treatment is provided, the aims are simple and clear. The requirements for success in endodontics are:

- understanding the role of microorganisms in the disease process;
- identifying microbial routes of entry into teeth;
- practising good infection control and disinfection procedures;
- the elimination of microorganisms from the pulp spaces of teeth;
- preventing re-infection of the pulp space by providing effective barriers to bacterial re-entry.

Disinfection and sealing of teeth are the essential components of treatment. The removal of organic nutriment, which is likely to support bacterial growth, although not a specific goal, is also important.

Thorough disinfection procedures are always accompanied by the need for complete coronal sealing to limit re-infection. During all treatment phases, this is achieved using provisional restorations. Following completion of endodontic treatment (Fig. A1.3) a well-fitting definitive restoration should be constructed as soon as possible to satisfy this requirement.

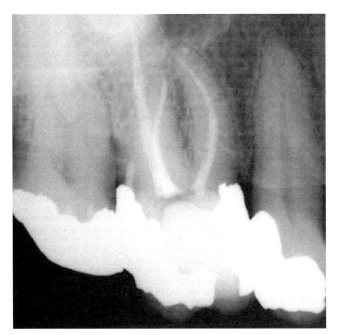

Fig. A1.3 Completed root canal treatment—a definitive coronal restoration is now required.

What does it take to be competent?

Endodontics is a clinical discipline that requires the development of a high level of diagnostic and clinical skills. You, as the student of the subject, will be required to reach a level of competence from which, in the long term, a higher understanding of the practised approaches to the delivery of care can flourish.

A number of countries now recognize endodontics as a specialty. Expertise in the delivery of care is exemplified by the standard of endodontic treatment expected of a specialist. The majority of endodontic treatments are and will continue to be provided by general dental practitioners and sadly, recent studies have indicated that the standard of endodontic practice carried out by general practitioners in Europe is not high.

In an attempt to improve and maintain standards of care for patients, it is appropriate to ensure that all students attain a level of competence prior to graduation. Through an ethos of continued learning and practice, all dental professionals have the opportunity to become more skilled.

Competence can only be attained through education and concerted training. The training needs to be competency based and practical skills experience should be gained in all areas of emergency and definitive endodontic management as related to total patient care.

The acquisition of basic skills is fundamental to future performance but can only happen gradually. Experience should be gained using models and extracted teeth as well as clinical cases. Laboratory and clinically-based practical skills should be monitored by experienced practitioners who themselves display a high level of ability. Quality assessment criteria and positive feedback are essential to the promotion of confidence and a sense of accomplishment. Intrinsic to the process of improvement is the development of accuracy in the use of criteria in the practice of self-assessment.

With the introduction of clinical governance by the UK Government, all dental practitioners will be accountable for continuously improving the quality of their services and safeguarding a high standard of care. Dentists and dental practices will be expected to be able to prove the following:

- clear lines of responsibility and accountability within which there is a comprehensive programme of quality improvement;
- clear policies aimed at reducing risks;
- procedures for the identification and remedy of poor performance.

The key elements of this governance will focus on the following:

- *Quality improvement processes*: every member of staff will need to recognize their role in improvement. Methods of improving care need to be identified. Dentists should be meeting patients' agreed and reasonably explicit expectations. To achieve this they need to consult and listen carefully to patients and staff;
- *Risk reduction*: by carrying out a risk management programme;
- *Continuing professional development*: to maintain personal standards.

With the introduction of a mandatory recertification scheme (for example, by the General Dental Council in the UK), all practitioners will be required to fulfil professional development requirements and continuing education to keep up to date with modern trends.

The maintenance of quality and standards in the provision of endodontic care will also require that all operators should aim for a level of achievement that represents all aspects of 'best practice'.

Competency in endodontics requires the use of two essential tools in the fight to reduce the endodontic microbial flora. These are the effective delivery of disinfecting agents and a means of efficient isolation of the operating field and the teeth. Rubber dam isolation should be considered a mandatory barrier for all cases and during all

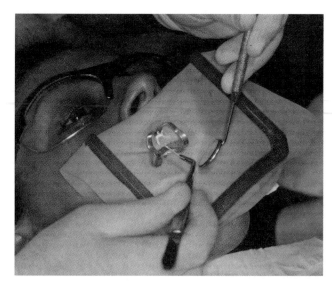

Fig. A1.4 Rubber dam in use during endodontic treatment.

stages of treatment (Fig. A1.4). Failure to employ rubber dam is contrary to acceptable standards. Rubber dam improves access and vision, reduces the risks to patients, controls infection and moisture, and increases operator efficiency. Most of all, rubber dam prevents the contamination of teeth by saliva and protects the patient's pharynx from the effects of the disinfectant. It is significant that the use of rubber dam was described long before microorganisms were identified as the cause of periradicular disease.

Competence in endodontics is hampered by the lack of acceptance of the use of rubber dam among UK dentists. Failure to employ rubber dam deters the use of potent but unpleasant disinfectant agents. It is not surprising therefore to find that the majority of dentists who fail to use rubber dam as a barrier also prefer to wash teeth out with local anaesthetic solution or saline rather than an acceptable and effective disinfectant.

In the last 25 years an increasing number of dentists have restricted their practice to endodontics. There has been a marked increase in the number of practitioners claiming registered specialist status in the UK. There is now a prescribed specialist training pathway for those wishing to become endodontists. The number of patients referred for specialist endodontic care continues to rise. This, and the tendency for patients requiring extensive treatment to receive integrated care, may well lead to improved standards of service.

How has the discipline developed?

Endodontal diseases have been well chronicled and there is evidence of both the suffering caused and the treatment methods employed to relieve pain over many centuries.

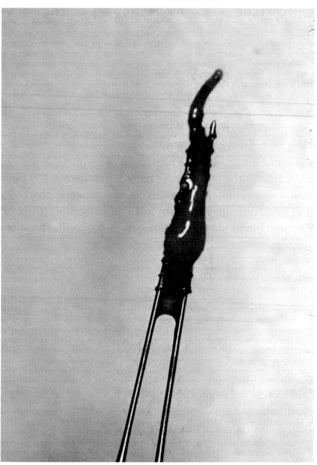

Fig. A1.5 An extirpated dental pulp.

Treatment to relieve pulpal pain has generally involved tooth extraction or removal of the dental pulp (Fig. A1.5).

The ancient Chinese believed that the tooth worm was the cause of dental caries and toothache. Early inscriptions from the fourteenth century BC have been located depicting the characters for both the worm and the tooth. Early treatments were aimed at reducing pain and putting the inflamed dental pulps, which were often the cause of the toothache, out of their misery. The topical use of arsenic and hot needles was common. In the Middle Ages people generally suffered the various chronic disorders without treatment and it was not until the eighteenth century that extraction became the means by which both dental pain and infection could be eradicated. Extractions were performed without local analgesia up to the end of the nineteenth century.

It is only in the last 150 years that microorganisms have become associated with the aetiology of endodontic disease. Miller (1894) first demonstrated the presence of bacteria in samples retrieved from the pulp spaces of teeth. The discovery of X-rays by Roentgen in 1895 increased the popularity of early attempts at endodontic treatment. However, when Hunter (1911) made his now famous pronouncements about the systemic effects of dental sepsis, dental radiography was used to champion the cause of the believers in the theory of focal infection. This led to extraction becoming the treatment of choice for periradicular disease, which handicapped the development of root canal treatment provision for the next 30 years.

The wheel seems to have moved full circle in the last 80 years and a small group of dental practitioners are returning to the ideology of the original theory; it is clear that the possible links between oral disease processes and systemic illness require fuller investigation. Current research hints that the existence of a relationship between standards of oral health and cardiovascular disease should not be ignored. It has been suggested that bacteraemias induced during endodontic treatment may also lead to potential systemic problems. Further research, involving controlled patient groups, is required to establish such links.

The post-Second World War years saw a resurgence of interest in endodontic practice. The American Association of Endodontists was formed and 20 years later the British Endodontic Society appeared on the scene. There are now, worldwide, more than 30 national and international bodies devoted to and interested in promoting the subject. This is testimony to the rapid development of endodontic practice.

The significance of microorganisms in endodontal disease was revealed in 1965. Normal rats developed disease when dental pulps were exposed to microorganisms. Gnotobiotic (germ-free) rats failed to develop endodontic infections following dental pulp exposures. Serious attempts at disinfecting teeth have been developed over the past 60 years. Treatment has involved the opening up of the root canals of teeth followed by attempts to eliminate microorganisms by delivering combinations of disinfectant solutions and medicaments to the interior of the teeth. At one time it was recommended that root canals be cultured to identify the microflora responsible for the infection. Culture techniques were unreliable and it was shown that the success rate for negative-cultured canals was no better than for those with positive cultures. It has only relatively recently been proved that a careful aseptic technique can lead to elimination of the microflora of teeth and consequent return to health.

Recent developments have seen the introduction of new materials, instruments, and equipment. The use of biocompatible Mineral Trioxide Aggregate (MTA) as both a pulp capping agent and a retrograde root-end filling material is an example of a material development. The physical properties of nickel titanium hand and rotary instruments have been studied and improved considerably. The increased use of digital radiographic equipment and operating microscopes stresses the technological advancements in this clinical area. Above all, the present understanding of the microbiological processes affecting teeth has led to the introduction of single use instruments and an appreciation of the infection control requirements of endodontic practice. Natural growth factors harvested from dentine matrix are being studied with the prospect of encouraging dentine formation and replacing essential components of the pulp–dentine complex.

What is the purpose of this text?

Endodontics is probably one of the most satisfying clinical disciplines within dentistry. It combines inquisitive and practical skills, which, if correctly applied, usually lead to predictable clinical outcomes. Pain of endodontic origin is the most common of all the pain problems presenting in the oro-facial region. An understanding of the causes of endodontal disease, coupled with effective clinical skills affords an operator the opportunity to relieve pain and conserve and retain teeth that might otherwise be extracted. The success rate for endodontic procedures is high and proficiency in this clinical discipline brings rewards to both practitioners and their patients.

Clinical endodontics in the UK has been traditionally taught as a part of conservative dentistry. There may be historical reasons for this. Conservative Dentistry normally concentrates on the restorative requirements that are necessary to deal with the destructive sequelae of dental caries, tooth surface loss, and trauma. Endodontics involves the treatment of infections of the pulp space and periradicular tissues that are also usually the result of invasion of microorganisms following loss of integrity of the teeth.

Traditional undergraduate courses in endodontics have, in the past, followed a pattern of lectures, practical demonstrations, and student practice. The teaching tended to be didactic and emphasized in a prescribed way 'how' rather than 'why' treatment is performed. Thankfully, the introduction of philosophies such as problem-based learning and student self-assessment procedures has heralded the introduction of new courses based on independent learning, which reflect the requirements for accurate judgement of standards of patient care.

The body of knowledge that represents endodontology has expanded enormously over the past 20 years. Basic research has improved the understanding of the microbiological and immunological aspects of the disease processes. Advances are being made at a rapid pace and modern technology has led to the development of sophisticated treatment apparatus. New approaches to treatment are the results of technically based research aimed at making root canal treatment a more efficient treatment modality but it could be argued that many of these new approaches fail to give full consideration to the biological aspects of treatment. A deep understanding of basic biological principles is required if recently introduced innovations are to be recognized and introduced into mainstream practice and clinicians are to adapt to future changes.

Living in a consumer-driven society, members of the dental profession are becoming aware of the pressures that are now being placed upon them to perform to high standards. There has been an increase in the awareness of the benefits of dental care and the expectations of patients have reached new heights. Failure to meet those expectations leads inevitably to mistrust and litigation. Today, the profession is expected to provide a quality service and remain current in all aspects of clinical performance; to this end, it needs to conform to the objectives of evidence-based best practice in order to progress the interests of modern oral health care procedures.

This book has been produced primarily for undergraduate students who wish to develop an understanding of what constitutes the basis of effective modern endodontic practice.

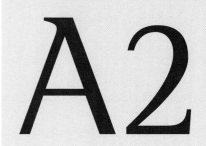

The life of a tooth

The life of a tooth

Introduction

In order to maintain acceptable standards of dental health care delivery, a sound knowledge of the anatomy, physiology, and pathology of teeth is an essential prerequisite for the practice of endodontics. An appreciation of the form and function of teeth assists greatly in understanding the disease processes that affect teeth during the course of a lifetime. There are many excellent standard texts that deal in detail with the anatomy, physiology, pathology, and microbiology of teeth. This chapter presents a view of those aspects of basic science that are particularly relevant to endodontics.

How does a tooth form?

The formation of teeth is a complex process, which involves interaction of the various tissues of the tooth bud (i.e. epithelial cells of the dental lamina) and the mesenchymal tissue of the dental papilla (Fig. A2.1).

The cells of the internal enamel epithelium and the dental papilla are separated by a basement membrane. The enamel-producing cells (ameloblasts) differentiate from the internal enamel epithelium. As they become differentiated, changes take place on the other side of the basement membrane within the dental papilla. Initially, a row of pre-odontoblasts form in the dental papilla adjacent to the basement membrane. This preodontoblast layer differentiates into odontoblasts—these cells produce dentine. *Odontoblasts* are highly specialized cells. They are post-mitotic end cells, which means that they no longer have the capacity to divide. Odontoblasts are responsible for matrix formation and mineralization of the dentine.

The mitotic activity of the internal enamel epithelium, interacting with the mesenchymal tissue of the dental papilla, produces the crown shape. Dentine matrix formation is first seen in the areas of the cusp tips. With the commencement of dentine formation the dental papilla takes on the role of the dental pulp.

Root formation commences with the downgrowth of Hertwig's epithelial root sheath, which is formed by the apical proliferation of the fused layers of the internal and external enamel epithelium. Through a process of continued proliferation, infolding, and differentiation, the root form of single- and multi-rooted teeth is delineated. The innermost layer of the sheath is responsible for the production of the root covering of cementum. The separation of the dental papilla from the surrounding mesenchymal tissue leads to the differentiation of the pulpal and periradicular tissues. Where there is a break in the sheath and separation is incomplete, neurovascular connections remain between the tissues. These connections persist throughout life as the apical, lateral, and accessory canals (Fig. A2.2). It should be emphasized that the pulpal and periradicular tissues remain intimately related at a neural and vascular level throughout life.

The crown and root forms of teeth are highly heritable and there are established genetically determined diversities in the dental form of modern human populations. For example, children tend to develop teeth similar in form to those of their parents and teeth are usually replicated on opposite sides of the dental arches as mirror images of each other.

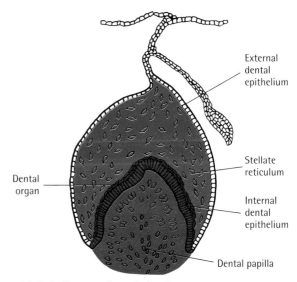

Fig. A2.1 Bell stage of tooth development.

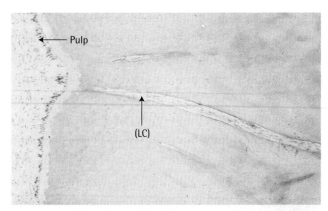

Fig. A2.2 A lateral canal (LC) demonstrated histologically.

An appreciation of the development, form, and internal anatomy of teeth is fundamental to the prevention, diagnosis, and treatment of endodontal disease. Changes take place to the internal anatomy of teeth as they develop and age. It is very useful to understand and have at hand calcification times, eruption dates, and apical root closure dates (Fig. A2.3).

Congenital malformations and aberrations should also be borne in mind (Fig. A2.4(a) and (b)). The development of teeth may be affected by conditions such as invaginations, evaginations, congenital grooves, enamel pearls, enamel spurs, talon cusps, dilacerations, and geminations.

What are the significant features of the dental tissues?

The primary and adult dentitions of humans have their own characteristics but can be schematically represented and divided into four recognizably different structures. These are the dental enamel, cementum, dentine, and dental pulp (Fig. A2.5). The tooth can be divided into the anatomical crown and root. The cervical or neck region of the tooth forms the natural divide between the two. The crown is covered with enamel, whilst the roots are covered with cementum. Within the body of the tooth there is the soft dental pulp housed within the body of hard dentine.

Dental enamel forms the protective outer layer for the crowns of teeth and the natural integrity of teeth depends upon its presence. It is the hardest of all the human tissues, having a highly mineralized structure consisting of over 95% inorganic matter by weight. The structure of the enamel is prismatic in nature, consisting of millions of hydroxyapatite crystals. Although a very dense material, enamel is permeable to certain ions and molecules and is liable to fracture. Moisture can also exude from enamel and dry enamel takes on a more opaque appearance. Small cracks or infractions are often observable within enamel (Fig. A2.6) and present a potential avenue for the entry of microorganisms into the pulp–dentine complex.

Tooth	Eruption	Crown maturation	Root maturation
All first molar and lower central incisors	6-7 years	3-4 years	9-10 years
Upper central incisors and lower lateral incisors	7-8 years	4-5 years	10-11 years
Upper lateral incisors	8-9 years	5-6 years	11-12 years
All canines	9-10 years	6-7 years	12-13 years
All first premolars	10-11 years	7-8 years	13-14 years
All second premolars	11-12 years	8-9 years	14-15 years
All second molars	12-13 years	9-10 years	15-16 years
All third molars	17-22 years	14-19 years	20-25 years

Fig. A2.3 Eruption and tooth completion dates.

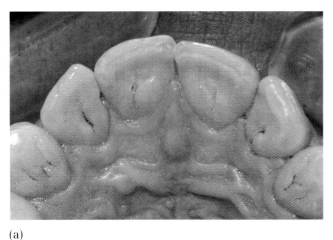

(a)

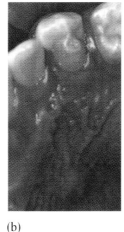

(b)

Fig. A2.4 (a) Deep cingulum pits in maxillary incisor teeth; (b) congenitally malformed maxillary canine with associated palatal sinus.

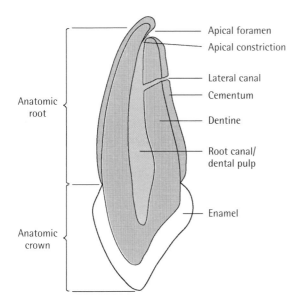

Fig. A2.5 Structure of a tooth.

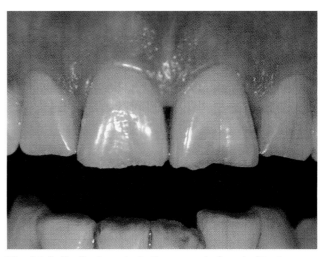

Fig. A2.6 Vertical cracks in the enamel of central incisors.

Cementum covers the surface of the roots and provides a means of attachment to the alveolar bone by way of the periodontal ligament. Sharpey's fibres form an attachment for the principal fibres of the periodontal ligament in the cementum. Two types of cementum have been identified. 'Acellular' cementum is located on the coronal half of the root surface and 'cellular' cementum is found on the apical half of the root surface. Cementum is laid down throughout life and, particularly in the apical region, can compensate for occlusal wear and eruption. It is worth remembering that cementum is permeable to a number of materials that may gain access to the dentine through the root surface. Loss of cementum leads to exposure of the underlying dentine. It is not uncommon for cementum to be damaged or removed during dental instrumentation

(for example, subgingival periodontal instrumentation). This then leads to the exposure of patent dentinal tubules.

Dentine forms the bulk of tooth structure and that covered by enamel is termed coronal dentine. The roots are made up of radicular dentine, covered by cementum. Dentine has a tubular structure, spanning its entire width from the dentino-enamel and dentino-cemental junctions to the pulp. In healthy teeth the honeycombed structure (Fig. A2.7) is bathed in tissue fluid from the pulp. It is more resilient than enamel but harder than either cementum or bone. Dentine is yellow in appearance, less reflective to light than enamel, and is only one-fifth as hard as enamel.

The *dental pulp* consists of connective tissue that occupies the pulp space or pulp cavity, which is surrounded by the dentine. The dental pulp and the pulp space tend to

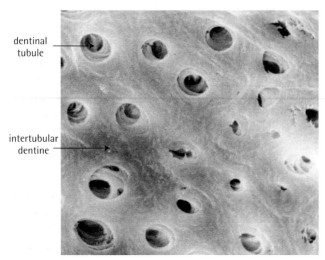

Fig. A2.7 Honeycombed appearance of dentine.

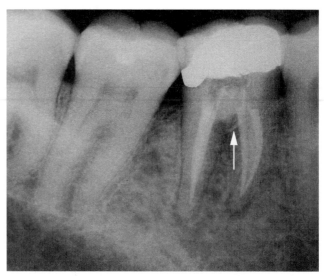

Fig. A2.8 Radiograph of root-treated molar tooth with lateral canal communicating with furcal region.

conform to the general shape of the root and they are divided into the coronal and radicular pulp. The radicular pulp communicates with the periradicular tissues through apical, lateral, and accessory canals. Such communication has been found in the coronal and middle thirds of over half all molars. Accessory canals may also connect the coronal pulp with the interradicular tissues through the floor of the pulp chamber (Fig. A2.8). This may allow the interchange of inflammatory breakdown products between the pulp and periodontal tissues. The *pulp-dentine complex* is the term used to describe the dental pulp and the dentine that surrounds it (Fig. A2.9). The dentine-forming cells, the odontoblasts, intimately connect the dentine and pulp. The three components of the complex behave biologically as a single unit and are functionally interrelated. The presence of a normal pulp–dentine complex is important for the maintenance of a healthy tooth. The dental pulp consists of blood vessels, nerves, cells, and ground substance. An odontoblast layer is located within the pulp immediately adjacent to the predentine, beneath which is a central core of blood vessels surrounded by a cell-rich zone and a cell-free zone.

In the main, blood vessels enter the pulp through the apical foramina and branch out laterally towards the odontoblast layer and subodontoblastic region. Arteriovenous anastomoses (shunts) facilitate the movement of blood directly from and to the larger vessels, avoiding the capillary beds. This facility provides a significant response to the irritant action of physical, chemical, or bacterial stimulants. Capillary blood flow in the coronal portion of the dental pulp is twice the volume of that in the capillary bed of the radicular portion. The greatest blood flow is in

the pulp horns. The pulp is relatively incompressible as it is encased within a rigid case of dentine. This also means that the total blood volume in the pulp cannot be greatly increased. Consequently, any small change in blood volume (for example, in cases of pulpitis) may lead to a significant change in local pressure and it should therefore be clear that regulation of pulpal blood flow is critical to

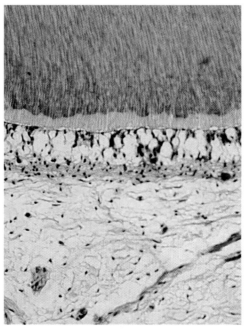

Fig. A2.9 Histological section of the pulp–dentine complex.

health. Local anaesthetic solutions may affect pulpal blood flow. It has been demonstrated that local anaesthetic solution containing adrenaline delivered by an intraligamental approach may severely reduce the pulpal blood flow. This in turn will affect the removal of metabolites and delivery of nutrients to the tissues. In the worst case scenario, the potentially toxic metabolites of an active pulp will accumulate and at the same time the pulp tissue will be deprived of essential metabolites (including oxygen) and inflammatory cells. Although this may not be significant in a healthy young pulp, it may be of critical importance in an already compromised tooth (for example, one that is already heavily restored).

The pulp has an exquisitely responsive sensory system. The thousands of axons entering a root consist of sensory myelinated low-threshold Aδ fibres (1–6 μm diameter), which respond to pulp testing, sensory myelinated Aβ fibres (6–12 μm diameter), which respond to touch and pressure, and sensory unmyelinated high threshold C fibres (0.4–1.2 μm diameter). C fibres are responsible for the transmission of slow, dull, less localized pain associated with pulpal inflammation.

The cells of the pulp include fibroblasts, undifferentiated mesenchymal cells, and macrophages. The most common cells found in the pulp are fibroblasts. They are very common in the cell-rich zone and are responsible for collagen and ground substance formation. The ground substance of the pulp is resilient, fibre reinforced, and helps limit intrapulpal pressure.

Dentine

The structure and function of dentine must be well understood. Dentinal tubules run from the pulp to the dentino-enamel junction, occupying 20–30% of the volume of the material. Dentine is less mineralized than enamel, with only 70% inorganic material by weight. There are up to 65 000 tubules per square mm at the pulpal end and 15 000 per square mm at the dentino-enamel junction. The diameter of the tubules becomes smaller from the pulp outwards. There are more tubules in coronal dentine than radicular dentine. The tubules contain tubular fluid, the long narrow odontoblastic processes of odontoblasts, and nerves (the odontoblast processes and nerves do not extend through the entire depth of dentine). The innermost layer of the dentine is called the predentine. It consists of unmineralized organic matrix and is approximately 15 μm wide.

The fluid found in the tubules is called tubular fluid. Tubular fluid occupies around 20% of the total volume of dentine and flows outwards from the odontoblasts and into the dentinal tubules. Fluid pressure of the pulp is approximately 10 mm Hg, which means that if tubules are open to the oral environment, the pressure gradient between the pulp and the external surface results in an outward flow of dentinal fluid. Antibodies and antimicrobial agents may be present within the tubular fluid of vital teeth. The coefficient of thermal expansion of the dentinal fluid is approximately ten times greater than that of the dentine.

Due to its tubular structure, dentine is permeable to fluids. Fluid permeation is proportional to tubule diameter and number. Dentine permeability therefore increases as tubules converge on the pulp. Radicular dentine is not as permeable as coronal dentine— it contains fewer tubules per unit area. The formation of dentine occurs throughout life (Fig. A2.10).

Primary dentine forms during tooth development at the rate of about 4 μm per day. *Secondary dentine* continues to be laid down over the entire pulpal surface once the tooth is fully formed. Its rate of deposition is about 0.8 μm per day. *Intertubular dentine* constitutes the bulk of the dentine (see Fig. A.2.7) (literally, dentine *between* the tubules). Its organic matrix is made up of collagen fibrils orientated at right angles to the dentinal tubules. *Peritubular dentine* is formed *within* the tubules during life. It is 40% more mineralized than other dentine and can lead to the occlusion of the tubules. *Tertiary dentine* is laid down in response to external stimuli at a rate of about 3 μm per day.

The terms *reactionary* and *reparative* tertiary dentine are often used to describe the response to localized potentially noxious stimuli. These stimuli include caries, tooth surface loss and restorative procedures. In addition to tertiary dentine, increased or accelerated deposition of peritubular

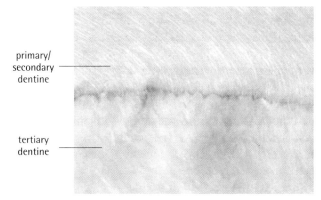

primary/
secondary
dentine

tertiary
dentine

Fig. A2.10 Histological section at the junction between primary/secondary dentine and tertiary dentine—the tubular structure becomes irregular.

(intratubular) dentine may occur. This hypermineralized dentine acts as another localized defensive barrier and results in accelerated sclerosis of dentinal tubules. The net result of the various types of tertiary and sclerotic dentine is to reduce the dentine permeability and increase the distance between noxious stimuli and the pulp.

These various defensive forms of dentine include the following:

1. *Reactionary dentine* is a localized dentine deposition laid down specifically in response to stimuli (usually low grade). The dentine secreted is from *existing* odontoblasts that created primary and secondary dentine. This tertiary dentine will have a similar composition to, and may be a continuation of, existing secondary dentine. The deposition of this form of dentine results in a distancing of the noxious stimuli from the pulp tissue.

2. *Reparative dentine* is laid down by *newly differentiated* odontoblasts and is usually stimulated by a severe injury, which damages the pulp–dentine complex and results in degeneration of existing odontoblasts. Because this dentine is being laid down by a new generation of odontoblasts, there is a resultant discontinuity of the tubular structure and therefore a reduction in dentine permeability. The reduction in dentine permeability may also be aided by a tubular hard tissue secreted by these new odontoblasts at the junction between the secondary and reparative dentine.

3. *Sclerotic dentine* involves the deposition of hypermineralized peritubular (intratubular) dentine by existing odontoblasts. This may be accelerated by localized stimuli and results in the reduction of the lumen size of tubules and therefore reduction in dentine permeability.

The quality and quantity of defensive dentine laid down is dependent on the status of the pulp and the nature of the injury. Low-grade irritation (for example, slowly progressing enamel caries) may result in mainly reactionary dentine deposition; however a more severe injury may result in the death of existing odontoblasts and secretion of less tubular reparative dentine from newly differentiated odontoblasts. All three types of defensive dentine may be present in different quantities depending on the severity and nature of the injury.

Dentine sensitivity can be explained by the 'hydrodynamic theory'. Aδ fibre nerves respond to deformation and fluid changes within the tubules. Any stimulus to dentine that extracts tubular fluid from the dentine results in stimulation of the Aδ fibres. For example, if dentine is stimulated with dry heat or air blasts, the resultant change in fluid pressure causes deformation of the odontoblastic process. This deformation is now thought to give rise to the release of a neurotransmitter substance, which activates the Aδ sensory plexus (also known as the plexus of Raschkow). The application of cold to dentine leads to tubular fluid contraction. Having a coefficient of thermal expansion 10 times greater than that of the tubule wall, the fluid contraction leads to Aδ fibre stimulation. Heat affects the tubular fluid by causing expansion. This in turn can raise the extravascular tissue pressure of the pulp.

The presence of mild inflammation in the pulp can alter the threshold of Aδ fibres. More severe inflammation gives rise to marked vasodilation and an increase in pulpal pressure. If the pressure exceeds the threshold of the unmyelinated C fibres, pain ensues (typically associated with the symptoms of irreversible pulpitis—see Chapter A3). The differentiation between the Aδ and C type of pain forms an important part of the diagnostic phase of care.

There is growing interest being centred on the role of the Aβ fibres in the protection of teeth. The fibres are sensitive to touch and pressure and may well offer protection to teeth by avoiding unnecessary trauma through a proprioceptive feedback mechanism.

As teeth get older they become less translucent and naturally darker. They also become less resilient and less permeable. The changes in the physical properties of the teeth are brought about by the continued production of secondary and tertiary dentine. A mechanism may well be at work to prevent the total obliteration of the pulp space and loss of physical resilience. It is known that secondary dentine formation occurs at a slower rate than primary dentine formation (0.8 μm per day instead of 4 μm per day). Aβ fibre transmission may well have an influence on the rate of dentine deposition, balancing the defensive role of deposition of the dentine against the loss of resilience of the tissue.

Other changes include reduction in pulp space volumes, a decrease in cell density and a reduction in vasculature, with a concomitant increase in fibrous tissue. These changes can result in a reduction in the ability of the pulp to recover from insult. Teeth also tend to become less sensitive as they age. There is a reduction in dentine permeability, which would seem to be a product of ageing and caries. The appearance of pulp stones and other dystrophic calcifications (Fig. A2.11) also contribute to physical changes within teeth and can make endodontic treatment more difficult.

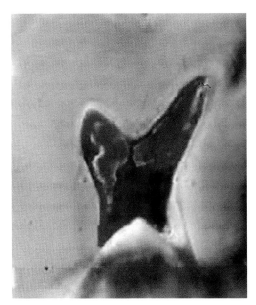

Fig. A2.11 Sectioned tooth revealing pulp stones (calcifications) within a pulp chamber.

What are the functions of the pulp–dentine complex in a mature tooth?

In addition to the general service performed by teeth in mastication and phonation, the pulp–dentine complex fulfils a number of specific functions throughout life. These functions are described as being those of dentine formation, maintenance, defence and propioception.

Dentine formation

The main function of the pulp–dentine complex in a mature tooth is the formation of dentine.

Maintenance

An intact blood supply is essential to ensure that all the necessary nutrients are delivered to and metabolites are removed from the cells of the pulp–dentine complex (for example, odontoblasts and fibroblasts).

Defence

The defensive role of teeth is probably underemphasized. Within the pulp–dentine complex, tubular fluid, peritubular dentine, secondary and tertiary dentine, and pulpal inflammation all play a role in the defence of the tooth. The stimulation of tertiary dentine production and pulpal inflammation can only occur within a healthy pulp.

Propioception

It appears that non-vital teeth may lose priopioceptors located within the pulp–dentine complex and this may result in tooth fracture when teeth are loaded during function.

In order to diagnose and deliver appropriate care for patients it is necessary to understand the basic mechanisms of dentinal pain, pulpal pain, dentine permeability and pulp testing. In healthy teeth, the pulp–dentine complex plays a crucial role in maintaining an environment within which the various described functions are sustainable. Should the viability of the pulp–dentine complex be lost, the functional capabilities of the pulp–dentine complex are also lost. Such teeth are no longer able to react to changing circumstances and must be considered indefensible.

What keeps a tooth healthy?

Teeth remain healthy by resisting disease. Endodontic reactions depend upon the virulence of microorganisms, the viability of the pulp–dentine complex and the immunological health of the host. The diseases that affect dental tissues are caries and periodontal disease. Over 350 different microorganisms have been identified in the oral cavity. The role of these organisms in the formation of dental plaque is well understood and their removal is an essential control measure in the prevention of these diseases.

Periodontal disease is caused by the accumulation of plaque in and around the gingival sulcus. The clinical picture varies from person to person and site to site. The disease may present as nothing more than a persistent gingivitis or may result in severe destruction of the periodontal tissues. The reason for this is that individuals show wide variations in their *susceptibility* to periodontal disease, which may be due to imbalances between the invading microorganisms and the immunological defence mechanisms of the host. Secondary factors, which locally affect the invasion potential of the microorganisms, or systemically affect the ability of the host to respond to the disease state, are significant to the clinical presentation. Local secondary factors include plaque traps (for example, carious cavities, overhanging margins, and partial dentures) and decreased antibacterial action of saliva. Systemic secondary factors include those of a genetic, infective, hormonal, haematological, and nutritional nature (for example, pregnancy, the effects of anticonvulsant drugs, and diabetes).

Endodontal disease is not unlike periodontal disease and represents an imbalance between the microbial invasion of the pulp–dentine complex or root canal system and host defence. The capacity of certain organisms to produce disease in a particular host depends upon the balance between the bacterial invasion and the viability of defence mechanisms of the host. Secondary factors, which locally affect the invasion potential of the microorganisms, or systemically affect the ability of the host to respond to the disease state, are significant to the clinical presentation. The tissues that constitute the pulp–dentine complex and periradicular tissues are able to react to the bacterial infections.

In summary, endodontal disease is the product of all aspects of microbial invasion, colonization, multiplication, and pathogenic damage to the teeth themselves. Disease outcomes depend upon the balance between bacterial attack and the state of the host defence mechanisms present at a particular point in time. The disease dynamics that occur in the pulp and periradicular tissues depend upon a number of factors that influence the balance between the bacterial attack and the host defence. These include:

- the state of the dental pulp and particularly the previous history of bacterial insult and tissue repair;

- the pathogenicity of the invading microorganisms;

- the duration of the insult;

- whether or not adequate treatment has been provided.

Teeth remain healthy when the balance of power remains tilted in favour of the host.

What threats do the oral microorganisms pose?

Where the balance of power moves in favour of the invading microorganisms, the nature of dentine and the dental pulp space is such that large quantities of microbes may be housed within the complex anatomy. The bacterial invasion of teeth can occur along a number of pathways. These include dentinal tubules, pulpal exposures, lateral and accessory canals and blood-borne routes. The tooth is naturally protected by enamel and cementum. Loss of these layers leads to the exposure of dentinal tubules. Consideration should be given to the variety of ways in which bacteria might enter teeth.

- *Caries.* In the early lesion, demineralization and the loss of continuity of the external surface of enamel leads to the loss of integrity of the tooth. Demineralization, bacterial penetration of dentinal tubules and destruction of dentine follow (Fig. A2.12a, b). The pulp–dentine complex's response to caries varies according to the rate of progress of the carious insult, the proximity of the lesion to the pulp and the status of the existing pulp. Carious, infected dentine does not have to be directly in contact with pulpal tissue to affect it. It has been shown that the pulp can be heavily inflamed even when the bacterial front is up to 0.5 mm from the pulp. Successful maintenance of pulp vitality at this stage will depend on the successful elimination of caries and prevention of further insults to the tooth.

- *Dental factors.* Whilst providing restorative care, dentists may damage reversible early lesions during the course of dental examinations by sharp probes. Operative and crown/bridge procedures also give rise to the unnecessary opening of dentinal tubules and, at times, accidental pulp exposures (Fig. A2.13a, b). Inadequate water coolant when using the air rotor handpiece and over-zealous drying of exposed dentine with a three-in-one syringe may result in pulpal damage. Inadequate isolation of teeth from saliva during such procedures can lead to contamination of the pulp–dentine complex. Bacterial invasion of the tooth is then facilitated. Failure to adequately protect and seal dentinal tubules increases the potential for microbial entry.

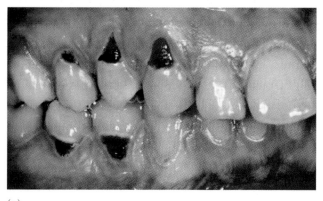

(a)

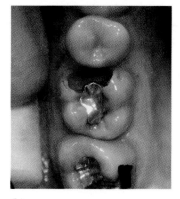

(b)

Fig. A2.12a, b
Established carious lesions.

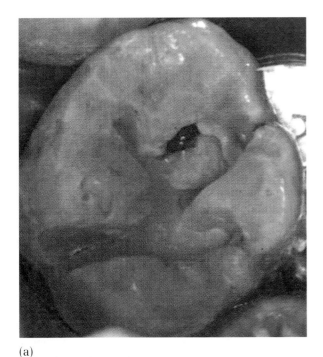

(a)

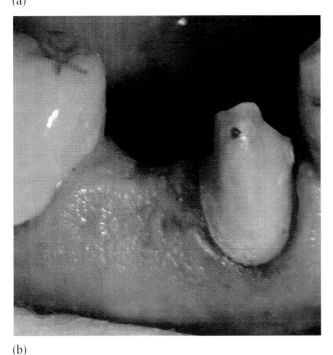

(b)

Fig. A2.13a, b (a) Cavity with freshly cut dentine tubules and accidental (mechanical) exposure; (b) Accidental exposure due to over zealous removal of dentine during crown preparation.

* *Physical trauma* can give rise to crown infractions, uncomplicated crown fractures, complicated crown fractures, and crown root fractures (Fig. A2.14). These

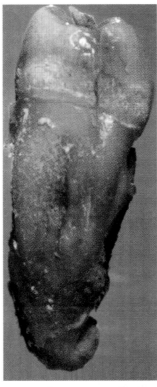

Fig. A2.14 Crown root fracture extending to the mid-third of the root surface.

conditions can all permit invasion of the pulp–dentine complex by microorganisms from the oral flora.

* *Tooth surface loss* (Fig. A2.15(a)–(c)), in the form of attrition, abrasion, erosion, and abfraction, also lead to crazes, patency of dentinal tubules, infractions and frank exposures of the pulp, which may result in the bacterial invasion of the pulp–dentine complex and finally the pulp. Premature ageing of the pulp, which occurs with long-standing or severe tooth surface loss, will also result in its reduced healing capacity.

* *Microleakage* is due to materials being poorly adapted to the tooth and this results in microscopic leakage of bacteria and their by-products between restorations and the cavity wall, leading to the pulp-dentine complex being affected (Fig. A2.16). Fluid may also permeate this interface and together with fluid within the dentinal tubules may act as a source of nutrient for existing bacteria trapped in the smear layer. The clinically undetectable penetration of microorganisms around restorative dental materials does more to promote damage to the dental pulp than the chemical effects of the materials themselves.

* *Periodontal disease and treatment* may also have an aggravating effect upon bacterial ingress into teeth. In

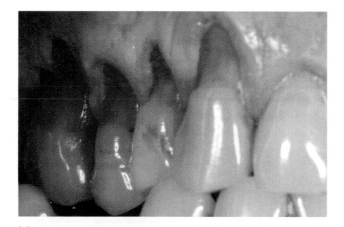

(a)

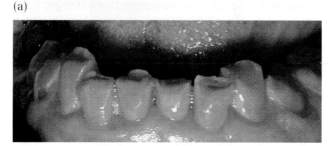

(b)

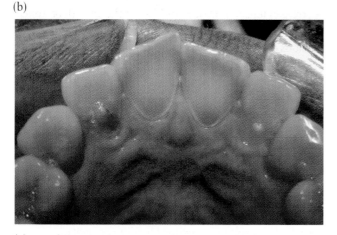

(c)

Fig. A2.15 (a) Tooth surface loss resulting primarily from abrasion; (b) tooth surface loss due to a combination of attrition and erosion; (c) palatal erosion resulting in hypersensitivity with cold liquids.

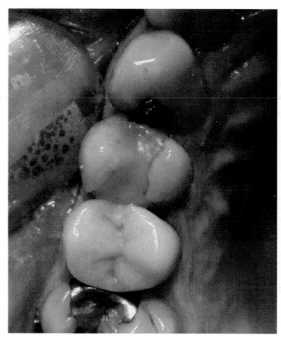

Fig. A2.16 Occlusal view of a composite restoration with poorly adapted margins which has resulted in pulpal symptoms due to microleakage.

As the microorganisms proliferate within the root canal system, tissue-damaging and inflammation-inducing products are in a position to diffuse freely through the tooth tissues. The bacterial by-products consist of enzymes and metabolic products, which have a direct toxic effect on the tissues. Certain components of the cell walls of the bacteria (endotoxins) also have the ability to induce inflammatory defence reactions. Short-term, low-grade irritation, if treated early, may lead to resolution. Long-term major insults can lead to inflammatory states that fail to resolve and may lead to pulpal necrosis and ultimately, periradicular pathosis.

The role of the oral microflora in pulpal and periradicular disease has been well documented. In a classical study, dental pulps exposed to the oral environment in germ-free rats were shown to have the capacity to heal, yet in normal, bacterially contaminated rats the pulps were unable to do so. Degeneration, inflammation and lack of calcific healing were evident. Many authors have confirmed the significant role of microorganisms.

Pulps that are overwhelmed by microorganisms or have had their vascular supply irreversibly damaged become necrotic. If microbes *infect* necrotic pulps there is the potential for the development of periradicular tissue reactions. It has been demonstrated that periradicular lesions only occurred in teeth where microorganisms were detected in their root canals. It has also been confirmed that periradicular diseases do not occur in *non-infected*, necrotic teeth.

theory, patent lateral and accessory canals that open into infected periodontal pockets may provide a route for the entry of microbes into the pulp–dentine complex. The removal of cementum during root planing procedures leads to exposure of dentinal tubules. Surgical procedures involved in crown lengthening and root resection may also lead to dentinal exposure and the potential for bacterial infection.

Periradicular pathosis is the result of a direct reaction between untreated root canal infection and host immunological defence mechanisms. The absence of a blood supply in the infected root canal makes it difficult for the body to fight the infection and, as long as the bacterial culture obtains nutriment, the infection persists (Fig. A2.17). Removal of the microorganisms from the tooth (or indeed removal of the tooth itself) leads to a process of healing and resolution of the periradicular lesion (Fig. A2.18(a)–(c)).

In intact teeth, endodontic infections are characterized by the presence of predominantly anaerobic microorganisms that live in the absence of oxygen. The infections are polymicrobial (multi-bacterial). Mixtures usually involve up to eight species. The microorganisms commonly isolated from an infected root canal system are *Prevotella* spp, *Porphyromonas* spp, *Fusobacterium* spp, *Peptostreptococcus* spp, *Eubacterium* spp, *Actinomyces* spp, and *Lactobacillus* spp.

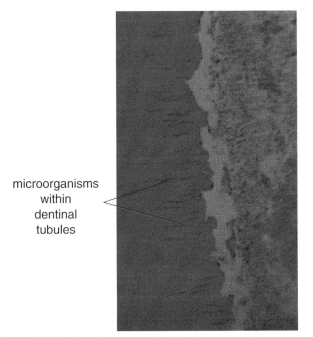

microorganisms within dentinal tubules

Fig. A2.17 Infected root canal with microorganisms penetrating the dentine.

Commensal, synergistic, and antagonistic relationships that exist between different species have been identified. These combinations of microbes and their products are responsible for tissue damage or immunological reactions. The actions of these bacteria and their products are largely the result of enzymatic activity. Bacterial enzymes accelerate the spread of the microorganisms, destroy defence cells of the host, and improve self-protection and attachment to tissues.

The toxicity of extracts of certain microorganisms has been confirmed. For example, *Porphyromonas* spp. are toxic to the cells of the dental pulp. They are also responsible for the release of protein-degrading enzymes, which have their effects upon immunoglobulins and mediators of inflammation. It is hardly surprising that extensive bone loss has been associated with periradicular infections involving the presence of organisms of this kind.

The ecological environment of the pulp space provides conditions that are favourable for the growth of certain microorganisms. Complex mixed flora can exist within teeth because:

- nutrients can be provided from disintegrating pulp tissue, saliva and inflammatory exudates;

- oxygen tensions are low and favour the growth of anaerobes (facultative anaerobes may occupy the coronal portions of the tooth where oxygen tensions are higher);

- bacterial interactions are favoured and exchange of nutritional products and the generation of necessary metabolites can take place.

Anaerobes need specific environments for growth to take place. This often takes the form of nutritional requirements provided by other microorganisms. This explains the association of mixed infections with endodontic disease. Particular combinations of specific organisms may therefore be associated with specific clinical presentations.

How are these threats resisted?

Saliva provides the front line defence to resist bacterial growth by constantly washing the surfaces of the teeth. It

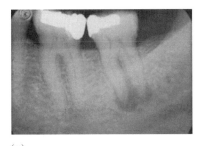

(a)

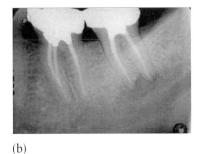

(b)

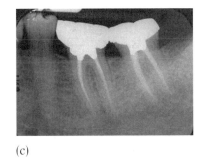

(c)

Fig. A2.18 (a) Radiograph of periradicular lesions associated with a mandibular molar; (b and c) radiographs showing resolution of the periradicular lesion following endodontic treatment 6 months following treatment (b) and 2 years following treatment (c).

also hinders the growth of bacteria by the action of certain specific and non-specific defence factors. These are bactericidal and fungicidal (for example, lysozyme and immunoglobulin A). It also has the ability to maintain pH by acting as a buffer.

The physical barriers provided by enamel and cementum also contribute greatly to the natural integrity of teeth. The impervious nature of enamel particularly resists the entry of microorganisms.

The pulp–dentine complex and periradicular tissues have the ability to react to insults of a microbial, physical and chemical origin. When these reactions relate to infection, they vary from mild inflammation to very severe and acute life-threatening conditions.

As previously mentioned, the outward flow of dentinal fluid resists entry of microorganisms. The tubular fluid also contains defence factors such as immunoglobulins, which also have a bactericidal action.

During various forms of dental procedures, including scaling, cavity preparation and root canal instrumentation, a smear layer is formed over the surface of the dentine. This smear layer (Fig. A2.19) is several microns thick and consists of a mixture of debris, bacteria (including their by-products), saliva, water and tubular fluid. The layer normally extends into the dentinal tubules. This closure of the tubules could be considered to reduce the permeability of dentine and offer a barrier to bacterial entry.

The permeability of dentine is also decreased by the process of sclerosis. This consists of continuing peritubular dentine formation and intratubular calcification. Peritubular dentine formation depends upon the presence of healthy odontoblasts whereas the intratubular calcification occurs when there is precipitation of mineral salts of previously dissolved calcium salts (Fig. A2.20).

Tertiary dentine formation (Fig. A2.21) also has a defensive role. It is laid down very rapidly and contains fewer dentinal tubules. It is formed in an attempt to compensate for dentine loss and provides a barrier that is more calcified than primary or secondary dentine.

In an attempt to dilute or neutralize the toxic effects of microorganisms the dental pulp can become inflamed. Inflammation is the body's response to potential and actual noxious stimuli. The aim is to protect the host tissue from damage. If damage does occur then it tries to consequently repair and regenerate the tissues. Inflamed tissues try to direct the body's immune system to that area. The response is organized into non-specific and specific

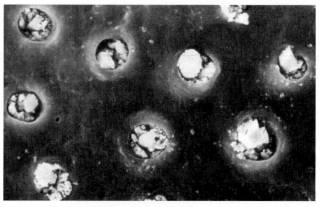

Fig. A2.20 Intratubular calcification—note the presence of crystals within the dentinal tubules.

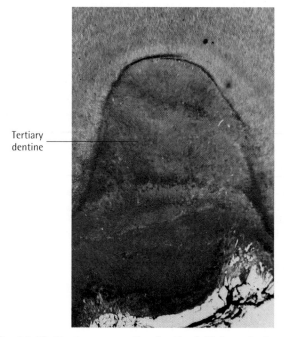

Tertiary dentine

Fig. A2.21 Tertiary reparative dentine laid down in the pulp space.

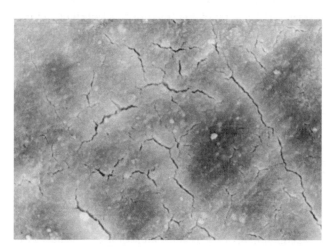

Fig. A2.19 Smear layer formation on the root canal wall.

responses. It is classically described as *calor (heat), rubor (redness), dolor (pain), tumor (swelling)*, and *loss of function*. Usually, pulpal inflammation is localized to the area adjacent to the source of noxious stimuli. An increased vascular permeability leads to loss of fluid from the vessels and increased tissue fluid pressure. The refined vascular structure of the dental pulp can divert blood away from the inflamed area while recovery takes place. In situations where the insult is very severe and the circulatory system is unable to compensate for the changes taking place, blood flow may cease and tissue destruction may give rise to tissue death or necrosis. This condition may gradually spread to involve all the dental pulp.

It should be emphasized that vascular impairment of the dental pulp plays a critical role in the progress of endodontal disease. The defence reactions of the pulp–dentine complex depend upon the presence of a healthy pulp. Total necrosis of the dental pulp leads to total loss of the natural defence mechanisms of the pulp–dentine complex. This in turn heightens the potential for the bacterial penetration of teeth. The difference in bacterial penetration of dentine in the vital and non-vital tooth has been demonstrated. Non-vital dentine is significantly more penetrable by invading microorganisms.

Once a tooth is restored, no matter how small the procedure, it is condemned to a spiral of periodic replacement of failing restorations—and potential damage of the pulp–dentine complex. Attention should always be paid to limit the amount of dentine exposed during restorative procedures to reduce the inevitable effects of microleakage.

What are the clinical outcomes of the disease dynamics?

The outcomes of endodontal disease are various and depend upon the many factors already referred to. The pulp–dentine complex may be affected by one entity or a combination. The diseases may be crudely divided into those principally affecting the dentine, pulp, and periradicular tissues. If the diseases affecting most superficial tissues are not treated or inadequately treated then they may progress and affect the pulp causing periradicular disease.

It is important to prevent damage to the pulp by either preventing disease, or if disease is present, by eliminating disease and preventing its recurrence. This may be achieved by either non-invasive approaches or, if invasive treatment is required, treatment modalities that cause the least harm to the pulp.

Pulpal conditions

Pulpal conditions are generally classified according to the presence of normal healthy tissue, inflammatory changes,

loss of pulpal tissue and degenerative changes. Inflammatory changes are described as being either reversible or irreversible.

- *Clinically normal pulp* is never spontaneously symptomatic. It is likely to respond normally to cold and electrical stimulation. Clinical examination and subsequent investigations are within normal limits. The radiographic picture of the pulp chamber, root canals and periradicular tissues is normal and consistent with the age and state of development of the tooth.

- *Reversible pulpitis* refers to the presence of mild inflammation in the pulp. The effects of this are such that the tooth might respond more than normal to stimuli (thermal and sweet) that tend to produce a short sharp pain. The pain resolves within 5–10 s after the stimulus is removed. Radiographic changes are not usually a feature, except if caries is visible on a bitewing radiograph. Once the cause of the inflammation (caries, leaking restoration, exposed dentine) has been treated satisfactorily, the pulp–dentine complex will return (*reverse*) to normal.

   Two further conditions that frequently affect the pulp–dentine complex are dentine hypersensitivity and cracked tooth syndrome.

- *Dentine hypersensitivity* presents as an exaggerated sharp, transient dental pain that cannot always be explained by common aetiological factors. It is usually a response to thermal, chemical, osmotic, tactile, or physical stimulation of exposed dentine. Stimulation of the exposed dentinal tubules causes fluid movement in the tubules, which results in the Aδ neural response at the pulp–dentine interface. Common causes include gingival recession and associated tooth surface loss (abrasion and erosion). Dentine hypersensitivity may be seen in patients who have received recent periodontal treatment, where dentinal tubules may become exposed. The aim of treatment is to identify and eliminate possible aetiological factors (e.g. vigorous tooth brushing) and to occlude or cover patent dentinal tubules (e.g. desensitizing toothpastes, varnishes and restorations).

- *Cracked tooth syndrome* patients usually complain of a sharp, shooting pain on biting hard objects. The pain may be difficult to localize. The symptoms are likely to occur on the release of the biting pressure (as the two cracked parts of the tooth come together); however, it may be difficult for the patient to identify this. The symptoms are again due to dentinal fluid movement transiently stimulating Aδ fibres. Once the 'cracked tooth' has been located, treatment is directed towards restoration with either cuspal coverage restoration (to keep the cracked tooth intact) or by replacing the cracked portion with a restoration. If this line of treatment is not successful then root canal treatment or, in intractable cases, extraction may be necessary.

♦ *Irreversible pulpitis* usually presents as a dull, throbbing ache (C fibre mediated pain) that lingers for minutes up to several hours. The symptoms may be spontaneous or initiated by temperature changes (for example, hot liquids). Patients may notice that the pain is worse at night or when they bend or lie down; this is due to an increase in intrapulpal pressure brought about by these postural changes. When periradicular inflammation is also present, the tooth may be tender to touch. The affected tooth may be difficult to localize and radiographic examination tends to be within normal limits. Radiographic changes are only recognized when the inflammation extends to the periradicular tissues. The pulp is referred to as being irreversibly inflamed on the basis that removal of the causal factor does not lead to recovery to a healthy state; if untreated the pulp will eventually become necrotic. The treatment options for irreversible pulpitis are root canal treatment or extraction.

♦ *Hyperplastic pulpitis* refers to the proliferation of pulpal tissue to produce a 'pulp polyp' (Fig. A2.22). It results from irritation usually associated with large carious exposures in young patients. The condition is usually symptomless and periradicular radiographic changes

are not common. Treatment options are root canal treatment or extraction.

♦ *Pulp necrosis* describes the death of pulpal tissue partially or totally as a result of loss of adequate blood supply. The necrotic tissue may not yet be infected, particularly if the condition was brought on by trauma that led to the severance of apical blood vessels. No radiographic changes are associated with the process of necrosis. The tooth will not normally respond to electrical and thermal tests. The necrotic tissue will eventually result in the development of periradicular periodontitis (see below); the tooth should either be root treated or extracted.

♦ *Pulp calcification* results in the obliteration of part or all of the pulp space due to an irritant stimulating the laying down of tertiary dentine. It is usually painless, unless it is accompanied by necrosis and bacterial infection. The crown of the tooth may be a darker yellow colour compared to the neighbouring teeth (due to tertiary dentine being deposited in the pulp chamber). Radiographically, there is partial or complete obliteration of the pulp space (Fig. A2.23). A periradicular radiolucency may be noted if the canals have become infected. Vitality testing is not always likely to produce a response. Electrical tests are more likely to elicit a reaction than thermal tests. Interventive treatment is indicated only if symptoms indicate irreversible pulpitis or there are radiographic changes indicating periradicular breakdown.

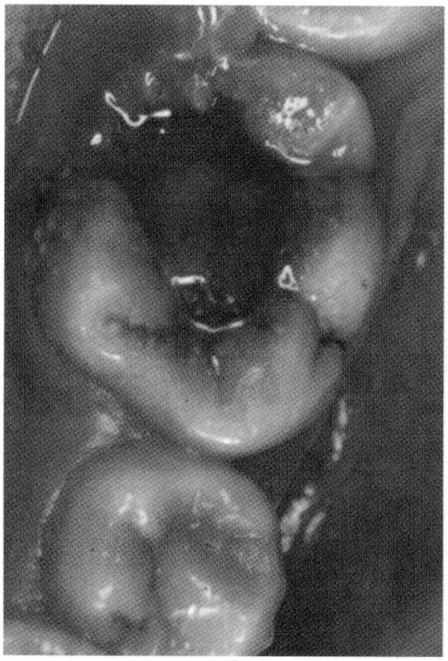

Fig. A2.22 Clinical example of hyperplastic pulpitis or 'pulp polyp'.

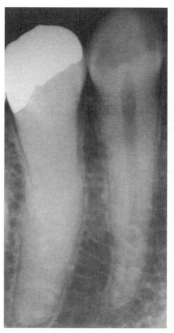

Fig. A2.23 Radiograph of mandibular premolar with a calcified root canal.

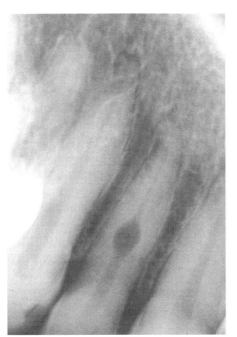

Fig. A2.24 Radiograph of lateral incisor with internal resorption.

♦ *Internal resorption* results in destruction of the internal aspect of the root canal by osteoclasts. It is usually an asymptomatic condition; thermal and electrical tests are unreliable. The radiographic appearance is one of a circumscribed round or oval radiolucency which is continuous with the root canal (Fig. A2.24). Immediate root canal treatment is the treatment of choice.

♦ *Periodontal–endodontal lesions* result from the intimate relationship that exists between the pulp and period-

ontal tissues. Periodontal lesions may develop around teeth that have infected pulp spaces. The pulpal infection spreads through the apical, lateral and accessory canals and drains via the periodontal ligamant (Fig. A2.25(a)). There should always be identifiable clinical and radiographic signs of pulpal necrosis and subsequent infection. Clinically, periodontal probing will reveal a deep, narrow, isolated pocket. The periodontal pocket is an extension of the endodontal disease process and therefore should resolve with the appropriate endodontic treatment (Fig. A2.25(b)). Periodontal lesions of periodontal origin have distinct probing patterns. They are usually wide and cone shaped. Radiographs reveal horizontal and vertical patterns of bone loss. Pain is not usually a feature and the status of the pulp remains normal.

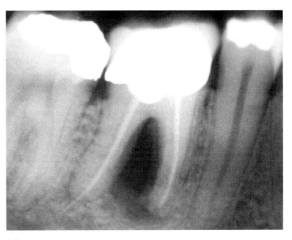

(a)

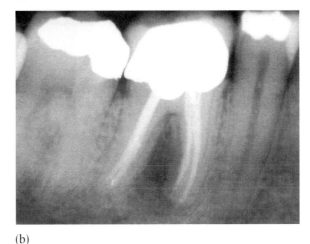

(b)

(a)   (b)

Fig. A2.25 (a) Endodontic infection giving rise to periradicular periodontal breakdown; (b) resolution of endodontal–periodontal lesion following root canal preparation alone. Note the absence of a root filling.

Fig. A2.26 (a) Previous root canal treatment in a mandibular molar with radiographic evidence of a periradicular and furcation lesion; (b) resolution of the lesion following retreatment.

Combined endodontal and periodontal lesions display concurrent problems in one tooth. An example of this is a *vertical root fracture*. Clinically, the fracture may or may not be obviously visible and separated. Deep, isolated periodontal pockets may be present adjacent to the fracture line and radiographs may reveal a localized radiolucency. The endodontal and periodontal lesions may or may not communicate. One lesion is due to pulp necrosis and subsequent infection, whilst the other lesion is an independent periodontal lesion. In time, and as the lesions develop, the origins of the processes become unclear.

♦ *Previous root canal treatment* could be considered to be an endodontic condition. The absence of a pulp and the presence of a root filling within a tooth does not negate the possibility of infection being present in the tooth (Fig. A2.26(a)). Retreatment, by removal of the existing root filling and accompanying infection, is required to promote healing (Fig. A2.26(b)). The recognition of early changes in the radiographic appearance of the periodontal ligament space may be crucial to establishing the likelihood of endodontic re-infection. Where periradicular lesions are evident radiographically, it is necessary to establish whether they are developing or perhaps resolving.

Periradicular conditions

Periradicular tissues include cementum, periodontal ligament, and alveolar bone. Periradicular periodontitis is the inflammatory disease of these tissues, which may be caused by *pulpal infection*. This inflammatory reaction is a response to *bacteria and their by-products* exiting the root canal system, mainly through the apical foramen. It is now known that altered host tissue, bacteria, and their toxins have the antigenic potential to initiate immune responses in the periradicular tissues. It is the host responses that account for much of the tissue damage. The term periradicular periodontitis is used in this text to describe the inflammatory conditions affecting the periradicular tissues. Traditionally, the term apical periodontitis has been used. Periradicular periodontitis is perhaps more appropriate because root canal systems are very complex and there are many potential avenues of communication with the periodontal ligament apart from the main apical foramen, which include the apical delta and lateral canals. Inflammatory change can therefore occur anywhere along the root including the furcation areas; thus the bacterial products can exit through any of these avenues causing inflammation periradicularly rather than just apically.

♦ *Clinically normal periradicular tissues* are found around teeth with normal periradicular health; these teeth are not tender to palpation or pressure and present with radiographically normal periodontal features.

♦ *Acute periradicular periodontitis* is the term used to describe acute inflammatory changes within the periodontal ligament. The condition is usually due to the presence of an infected pulp or occlusal trauma. Patients present with tenderness on biting. Clinical examination will reveal tenderness to vertical (and horizontal) percussion. The tooth may not respond to vitality testing and this would indicate pulpal necrosis. Radiographic thickening of the periodontal ligament space may be apparent. In early cases, however, the appearance is usually normal. Root canal treatment or extraction will be necessary in cases of pulp necrosis. If the symptoms are due to occlusal trauma, examination may reveal a high spot on a recently placed restoration and/or a positive response to vitality testing. Occlusal adjustment will be necessary if the diagnosis is occlusal trauma.

♦ *Chronic periradicular periodontitis* is due to an infected necrotic pulp. Teeth affected by chronic periodontitis may be symptomless or feel 'different'. Clinical examination may reveal mild tenderness to percussion or palpation or no response to vitality testing. Radiographs would show a radiolucent area associated with the roots of the tooth in question, reflecting the presence of granulomatous tissue (Fig. A2.27).

♦ *Chronic periradicular periodontitis with an associated sinus* refers to teeth which have the symptoms and signs of chronic periradicular periodontitis and in addition, examination reveals the presence of a sinus tract (Fig. A2.28). The sinus may be found intraorally or extraorally on the skin. Patients may complain of the presence of a gumboil, bad taste or smell. An obvious

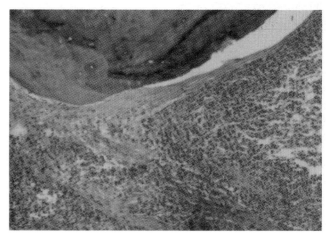

Fig. A2.27 Granulomatous tissue adjacent to an apical foramen.

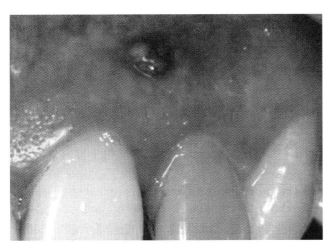

Fig. A2.28 A sinus tract associated with a discoloured lateral incisor.

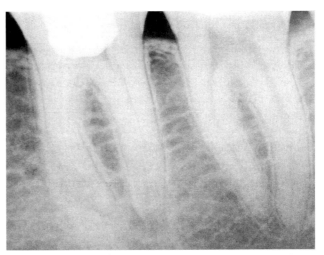

Fig. A2.30 Radiograph of condensing osteitis related to a mandibular first molar.

periradicular radiolucency will be apparent. Root canal treatment or extraction should be carried out.

♦ *Acute periradicular abscess* is a localized collection of pus, which occurs usually in the apical region of an infected tooth. The symptoms range from mild to severe pain and swelling. There is often tenderness to palpation and mobility of the affected tooth. There may be accompanying malaise, fever and lymph node enlargement. Intraoral and extraoral swelling may be present. Drainage of pus is an integral part of treatment for such conditions (Fig. A2.29) and antibiotics may also be required. Once the swelling resolves, root canal treatment or extraction may be carried out. The term *phoenix abscess* is used to describe this condition when it arises during the process of (re-) root canal treatment.

♦ *Condensing osteitis* is an easily distinguished condition where the radiographic appearance of the periradicular bone appears more radiopaque (Fig. A2.30). The pulp tissue of the tooth is chronically inflamed and may respond to thermal and electrical testing.

Pulpal conditions

♦ Normal pulp
♦ Reversible pulpitis
♦ Dentine hypersensitivity
♦ Cracked tooth syndrome
♦ Irreversible pulpitis
♦ Hyperplastic pulpitis
♦ Pulp necrosis
♦ Pulp calcification
♦ Internal resorption
♦ Periodontal-Endodontal lesions
♦ Previous root canal treatment

Periradicular conditions

♦ Clinically normal periodontium
♦ Acute periradicular periodontitis
♦ Chronic periradicular periodontitis
♦ Chronic periradicular periodontitis with an associated sinus
♦ Acute periradicular abscess
♦ Condensing osteitis

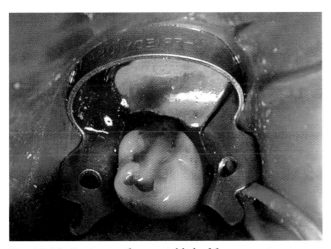

Fig. A2.29 Drainage of pus established for an acute periradicular abscess through the root canals.

Fig. A2.31 Common conditions involving the pulp and periradicular tissues.

Summary

The delivery of appropriate treatment and care for patients with endodontal disease requires a good working knowledge of the anatomy, physiology, and pathology of teeth. The conditions that result from the interaction of micro-organisms and their hosts require accurate identification before the appropriate treatment can be instigated. A knowledge of the basic science that underpins the disease dynamics is integral to the recognition and treatment of pulpal and periradicular disease (Fig. A2.31). Further, the disease process is dynamic and symptoms and signs may occur at many points on a 'sliding scale' of severity. This adds to the complexity of accurate diagnosis.

Diagnosis and treatment planning

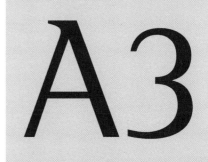

Diagnosis and treatment planning

What is diagnosis?

Diagnosis is a process by which a disease or abnormality is identified by collecting information about the presenting symptoms, clinical signs and the results of specific investigations. *An accurate diagnosis is the key to successful treatment.* The importance of the process cannot be overemphasized. The subsequent treatment options and planned management of the patient depends upon this diagnostic phase. It is necessary to arrive at a correct diagnosis even if this only means ruling out common dental disorders as being causative factors.

The question 'Is this a dental problem or not?' should always be asked. If the problem does not appear to be associated with teeth (odontogenic), it may be necessary to consider other causes of oro-facial pain (Fig. A3.1a). The clinician should always maintain a broad perspective when considering patient problems and the possibility of differential diagnoses should always be borne in mind.

In general, endodontic diagnosis involves identifying the extent of pulpal and periradicular disease in order to arrive at a suitable treatment plan. This plan should always take account of the patient as an individual, the difficulties that are likely to be encountered in the restoration of the tooth after endodontic treatment and the competence of the clinician. Some of the initial questions you should ask *yourself* are shown in Fig. A3.1b.

How do we arrive at a diagnosis?

A sound diagnosis can only be reached when information is systematically collected from the patient (Fig. A3.2). This information can then be interpreted and acted upon. Each step of the diagnostic procedure aims to (1) maximize the information gained from each stage of the diagnostic procedure before going onto the next and (2) help guide the clinician to the direction in which the next stage of the investigation should concentrate.

When the information from one aspect of the diagnostic procedure does not tally with the results from another

---

Musculo-skeletal pain
(e.g. temporo-mandibular dysfunction)

Neuropathic pain
(e.g. trigeminal neuralgia)

Neurovascular pain
(e.g. migraine, cluster headache)

Autonomic pain
(e.g. sympathetic nervous system mediated pain, atypical facial pain)

Psychogenic facial pain

Fig. A3.1a Common non-odontogenic aetiologies of oro-facial pain.

Is this an odontogenic problem?

Is this pulpal and/or periodontal pain?

Is this a healthy pulp or not?

Can I treat this individual?

Fig. A3.1b Questions that should be running through your mind when assessing the patient.

aspect of the diagnostic procedure(s) it can either mean that further investigations are required or that information that has been collected is insufficient or inaccurate.

Diagnostic errors usually occur when the clinical examination is incomplete, that is, one or more stages of the diagnostic procedure have been missed; when this occurs it can lead to the dentist going down the wrong avenue of investigation and, more crucially, towards formulation of an incorrect treatment plan.

---

(1) Patient history

Presenting complaint (reason for attendance)
History of presenting complaint(s)
Dental history
Medical history
Personal history (including social history)

(2) Examination of patient

General observations
Extra-oral
Intra-oral

(3) Special investigations

Vitality testing
Radiographic examination

(4) Differential diagnosis

Treatment options
Treatment plan

Fig. A3.2 The stages of clinical examination.

History taking

The aim of history taking is to gain an insight into the nature and character of the patient's symptoms and it forms the core of all aspects of clinical dentistry. This section focuses on aspects of history taking that are of direct relevance to endodontic diagnosis. The history, freely given by the patient, is a crucial part of the information gathering process. The operator will also be able to elucidate if there are contributory or aetiological factors in the patient's personal, dental, or medical history.

The history may also reveal potential complications or potential modifications to treatment planning, for example, if the patient has a phobia of dentists or has had a very bad experience at a previous visit. By gaining information from the patient the dentist will first be building a picture of the most probable causes of the patient's complaint(s) and thinking ahead about the main aspects of the extra- and intra-oral examinations and special investigations they may want to assess or confirm. Secondly, revelations from the patient's past dental history may mean that the operator may have to modify the approach (for example, rheumatoid arthritis may necessitate a different chair position and operator posture).

The amount of useful information obtained from the patient varies and depends on several factors. These include the patient's ability to convey or describe the symptoms that are being experienced, the degree of dental awareness demonstrated, the severity of distress/discomfort/pain at that moment, and the concern expressed by the patient. At times, a patient may present with more than one complaint. In these situations it is easier to concentrate on each complaint separately and prioritize them according to their seriousness.

Presenting complaint

Whilst establishing the reason for attendance it is possible to glean something about the patient's personality and attitude to dental treatment. Irrespective of the reason for attendance (that is, as an emergency, for routine examination, for a second opinion) opening questions should be simple and to the point. 'How may I help?' is an opening question posed by many dentists. The first few moments of listening to the patient are invaluable and may not only give an indication of the presenting complaint but also give an insight into their motivation and expectations. These expectations may or may not be realistic, desirable or achievable. Patients should be well motivated to undergo endodontic treatment. Poorly motivated patients should be encouraged to choose simpler forms of treatment.

History of presenting complaint

An attempt should be made to find out how long the patient has been suffering from their presenting complaint(s) and if/how the presenting symptom(s) has changed with time.

Dental history

Attendance

It is useful to know about the patient's previous dental history to establish whether they attend regularly, or only when in pain. If pain is the reason for seeking a second opinion, it is worth establishing whether the present problem is in any way related to recent dental treatment.

Oral hygiene and dietary habits

The patient's oral hygiene practices should be noted. The sugar consumption and acidic components in the diet should also be quantified. Key questions may help in finding the causal factors for the patient's complaints (see Chapter B3).

Previous trauma

It may be pertinent to ask if the tooth in question has been involved in dento-alveolar trauma. This scenario will occur more frequently in anterior than posterior teeth; for example, pulpal necrosis or discolouration of an unrestored anterior tooth may be explained by a previous dento-alveolar injury (such as from a sports injury or assault) (Fig. A3.3(a) and (b)).

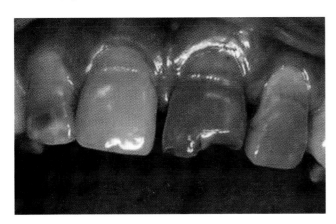

(a)

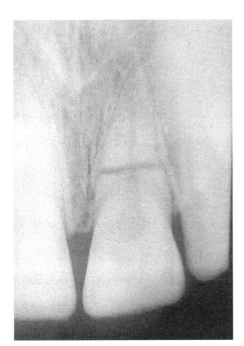

(b)

Fig. A3.3 The effects of trauma: (a) discolouration due to pulp necrosis; (b) horizontal root fracture.

Medical history

A thorough medical history must be taken and should also be regularly updated. The aim is to ascertain if there are any medical conditions or complications that may influence dental management. If there are any uncertainties or queries about the general health of the patient or if dental treatment may affect the patient, it is advisable to liaise with the patient's general medical practitioner or consultant.

Before prescribing any type of drug as part of the dental treatment, it is essential that the clinician checks whether there is a possibility of interaction with the medication that patients may already be receiving. A well-designed medical history form is a useful way of obtaining information. This becomes increasingly relevant with the increasingly complex drug regimes seen in an ageing population.

Common medical problems that may influence the diagnostic process or require the treatment plan to be modified include:

◆ susceptibility to infective endocarditis and the need for antibiotic cover (Fig. A3.4);

◆ hypertension;

◆ blood dyscrasias, anticoagulation therapy;

◆ recent history of a myocardial infarction;

◆ immunocompromised patients;

◆ steroid treatment (or recent history of steroid treatment);

◆ high-risk patients (for example, hepatitis B positive, HIV positive);

High risk:

◆ Prosthetic heart valve(s)

◆ Previous history of bacterial endocarditis

◆ Complex cyanotic congenital heart disease

◆ Surgically constructed systemic pulmonary shunts

Moderate risk:

◆ Acquired valve dysfunction (e.g. rheumatic fever)

◆ Most other congenital cardiac malformations

◆ Hypertrophic cardiomyopathy

◆ Mitral valve prolapse with regurgitation and/or thickened leaflets

Fig. A3.4 Antibiotic propylaxis is recommended for these conditions as they carry an increased risk of bacterial endocarditis.

♦ diabetes;

♦ history of depression or psychiatric problems;

♦ pregnancy;

♦ allergies.

For certain treatments, the patient's medical history may not be an issue. For example, the non-surgical endodontic treatment of patients taking anticoagulants should rarely present problems. However, there is an issue when such patients are required to undergo surgical procedures (extraction, periradicular surgery) and current guidelines must be followed. A note should also be made of any antibiotics (including dose, frequency, and duration) that the patient has recently taken, as this may influence the prescription of any further antibiotics that become necessary. Specific questions regarding allergy to latex (rubber dam and rubber gloves), household bleach and iodine (irrigants) should be asked as these materials and chemicals are commonly used in endodontic treatment.

Personal history

It is useful to obtain an insight into the patient's personal and professional lifestyle. This sometimes reveals clues to possible contributing or aetiological factors that might have a bearing on the presenting symptoms. A classic example of this is in individuals suffering from musculo-skeletal symptoms and signs (for example, temporo-mandibular dysfunction), initiated or aggravated by episodes of stress in their personal or professional life. These symptoms may be confused with endodontal disease affecting the pulp.

Extra-oral examination

The aim of the extra-oral examination is to look for signs of actual or potential pulpal or periradicular disease, for example, swelling or trismus and also to eliminate non-odontogenic causes of the patient's presenting symptoms.

Intra-oral examination

Access

Very early in any examination it is wise to establish whether there will be sufficient access to undertake endodontic procedures. Patients with restricted opening may be unsuitable for treatment particularly if access is required to posterior teeth (Fig. A3.5).

Brief general examination

The general state of the oral cavity should be surveyed before homing in on the area of the main complaint. This will give the operator an insight into:

♦ oral hygiene status (Fig. A3.6);

♦ caries level (Fig. A3.7 (a) and (b));

♦ how extensively restored the dentition is for the given age of the patient (Fig. A3.8 (a) and (b));

♦ the standard of (previous) professional oral care (Fig. A3.9 (a) and (b)).

This should then be correlated to the patient's past dental history.

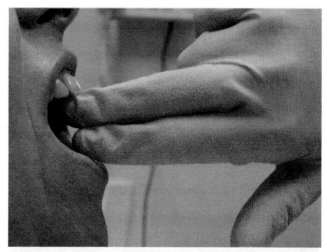

Fig. A3.5 Gloved hand gauging ability to open wide and accessibility for treatment.

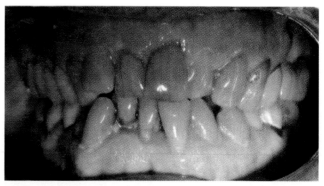

Fig. A3.6 A 62-year-old patient with poor oral hygiene; note the plaque accumulation at the gingival margins of the anterior teeth.

Detailed examination of the area of main complaint

A detailed examination of the area(s) of discomfort should be carried out. First, the area in question should be assessed visually; a note should be made of any abnormal appearance of the overlying mucosa (sinus tract, erythema, abscess) (Fig. A3.10).

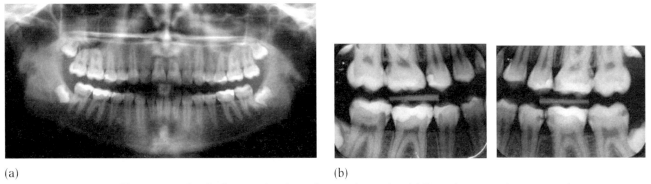

(a)   (b)

Fig. A3.7 A 17-year-old patient with a high sugar intake and extensive caries: (a) Dental panoramic tomograph; (b) bitewings.

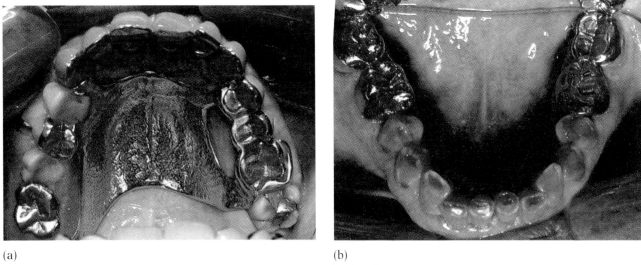

(a)   (b)

Fig. A3.8 (a and b) A 70-year old patient with a heavily restored and well-maintained dentition.

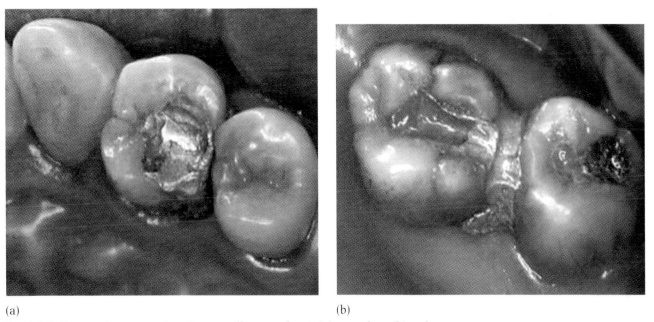

(a)   (b)

Fig. A3.9 Poor quality restorations in a maxillary quadrant: (a) premolars; (b) molars.

The next stage is to assess the alveolar region housing the tooth or teeth in question to assess the periodontal status, after which the teeth are examined. The following specific examinations should be carried out:

Palpation

Tenderness or swelling of the overlying mucosa usually indicates inflammation in the adjacent periradicular area, which has become extensive enough to break through the cortical plate.

Mobility

Excessive mobility may be due to clinical attachment loss as a result of chronic periodontal disease or an acutely inflamed periodontal ligament resulting from pulpitis or occlusal trauma (note that other common causes of excessive mobility include vertical/horizontal root fracture or decemented posts).

Percussion

This response indicates that the associated periodontal ligament is inflamed. This situation may arise from an

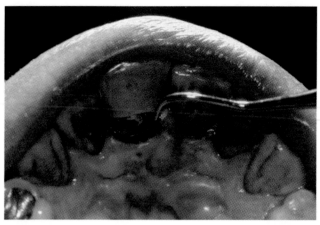

(a)

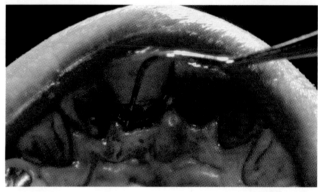

(b)

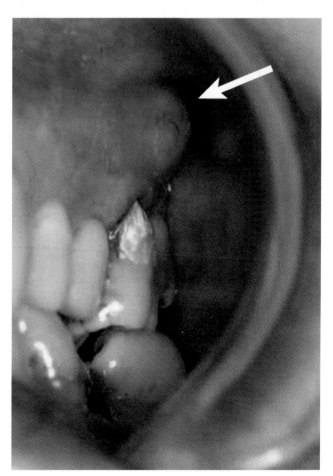

Fig. A3.10 Intra-oral swelling related to maxillary molar.

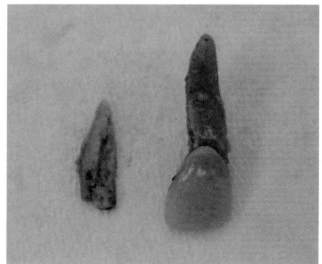

(c)

Fig. A3.11 Vertical root fracture in a post-crowned central incisor: (a and b) 'walking' a periodontal probe around the margins reveals a deep, isolated and narrow periodontal pocket adjacent to the fracture line; (c) fractured fragments following extraction.

infected necrotic pulp space. However, a common non-endodontic cause is occlusal trauma.

Periodontal probing

A detailed periodontal examination should be carried out on teeth under investigation. The ability to probe the furcation region of a molar may indicate the presence of periodontal disease. Conversely, if the tooth has undergone previous conservative or endodontic treatment, an iatrogenically induced perforation or vertical root fracture may be the cause of loss of attachment and increased periodontal pocketing. A localized deep periodontal pocket is commonly a sign of vertical root fracture (Fig. A3.11(a)–(c)).

Occlusal examination

Vital information may be elicited and help in the formulation of an accurate diagnosis, so do remember to include an assessment of the occlusion in your examination. It may reveal signs of occlusal trauma, parafunctional habits, or musculo-skeletal pain. This information may be important as occlusal disturbances may present with symptoms similar to pulpal or periradicular disorders. Undiagnosed occlusal trauma may ultimately lead to the propagation of cracks and fractures. These in turn may give rise to endodontic problems, such as cracked tooth syndrome or, by acting as an avenue for bacterial ingress lead to infection of the pulp space.

Assessment of teeth

The strategic nature of the tooth or teeth under investigation should be assessed as this may well have a bearing on the final treatment plan. For example, unopposed and non-functional teeth may well benefit from extraction.

It should be borne in mind that any breach of tooth structure indicates a loss of integrity of the crown and as such has the potential to initiate and perpetuate pulpal and periradicular disease. It is worth noting:

- crazing, infractions and fracture lines in the enamel (Fig. A3.12);

- primary and recurrent secondary carious lesions (Fig. A3.13);

- restorations with signs of microleakage or macroleakage (Fig. A3.14 (a) and (b)) (that is, ditching, open and discoloured margins) which act as plaque retention factors may lead to pulpal involvement (Fig. A3.15) and if large enough lead to food packing—this in itself has the capacity to mimic pulpal symptoms;

- Exposed dentine and pulpal tissue that may give rise to hypersensitivity or pulpal changes (Fig. A3.16); exposed pulpal tissues may be very obvious in some cases, for example, traumatized teeth (complete crown fractures) or gross caries but in other scenarios, pulp exposure may be more difficult to detect.

During clinical examination an attempt should be made to visualize the amount of sound coronal tooth that would remain after removal of caries and previous restorations. This may give a guide to the restorability of the tooth. Endodontic treatment is futile when carried out on teeth that are clearly unrestorable. When teeth appear restorable, the amount and position of remaining tooth tissue will influence the type of procedure performed for the construction of a post-endodontic restoration.

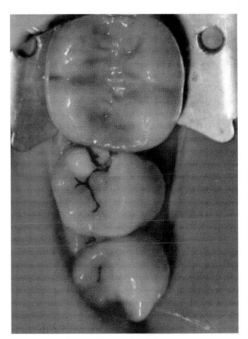

Fig. A3.13 Primary caries is the cause of irreversible pulpal change in this mandibular second premolar.

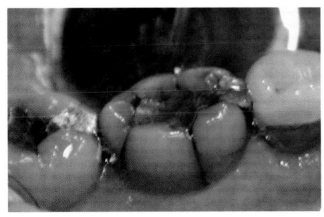

Fig. A3.12 Fracture lines in a molar tooth.

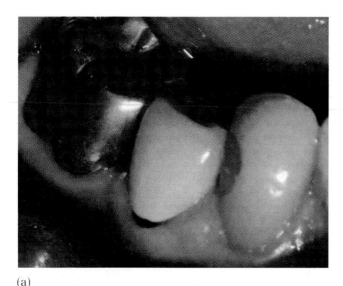

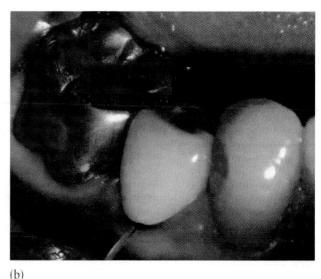

(a)   (b)

Fig. A3.14 (a) Suspect margin of crowned premolar; (b) probing around crown margins reveals deficiencies.

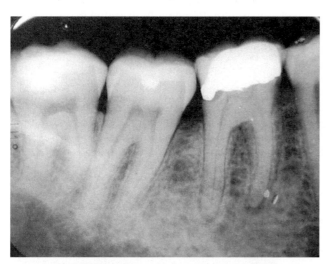

Fig. A3.15 Radiograph shows the route of infection at the distal margin of the crowned mandibular molar.

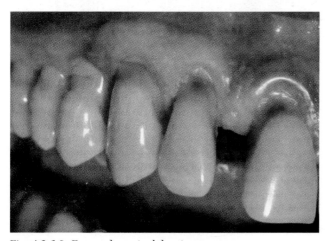

Fig. A3.16 Exposed cervical dentine.

The discolouration of teeth

This should also be noted (Fig. A3.3(a)). This discolouration may be due to one of many causes. Those of endodontic relevance include:

- pulpal haemorrhage;
- pulpal necrosis;
- microleakage;
- endodontic root filling materials in root-treated teeth.

Special investigations

The final stage in the assessment of the teeth is the use of special investigations, the commonest of which are vitality testing and radiographic examination.

Vitality Testing

The aim of vitality testing is to attempt to assess the health of the pulp. The tests that are commercially available assess crudely the responsiveness of the nerve supply only. It is assumed that the status of the nerve supply will also reflect the status of the blood supply (vascularity) of the tooth.

Electric pulp testing

This test involves the use of a battery-operated device to assess pulp vitality (Fig. A3.17). A positive response is usually due to the electric current stimulating Aδ nerve fibres. An indication of a healthy pulp–dentine complex is given when, on removing the stimulation, the sensation quickly disappears. When a lingering dull ache persists following the removal of the electric pulp testing probe it

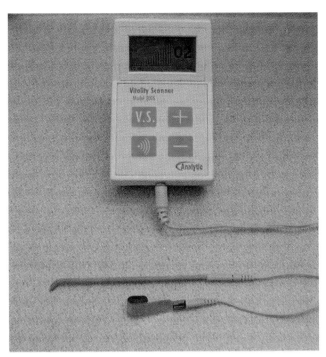

Fig. A3.17 Electric pulp tester (Analytic vitality scanner).

suggests that there has been stimulation of the C fibres, which is indicative of irreversible pulpal inflammation. No response from pulp testing indicates that the tooth is non-vital, that is, the pulp is necrotic.

Cold testing

Cold thermal testing can be performed using a number of agents (Fig. A3.18(a) and (b)). In teeth with healthy pulps Aδ nerve fibres are stimulated through the effects of contraction of the tubular fluid within dentinal tubules. Cold may relieve irreversible pulpitis pain by reducing the extravascular pressure within the pulp.

Heat testing

Thermal tests employing heat (Fig. A3.19(a) and (b)) can be performed to stimulate the Aδ nerve fibres in healthy teeth and may precipitate C fibre pain in irreversibly inflamed pulps. The types of responses that thermal tests produce are similar to those produced by electric pulp testing. An initial sensitivity that resolves soon after the stimulus has been removed from the tooth indicates the stimulation of Aδ nerve fibres. A lingering dull ache afterwards is indicative of C fibre activation, which may indicate irreversible pulpal changes. No response may be a sign of a non-vital tooth.

Test cavity preparation

It has been suggested that, as a last resort, a test cavity might be cut in a tooth without a local anaesthetic to establish vitality. Indiscriminate test cavity preparation is not advisable particularly when teeth are restored with expensive extracoronal restorations.

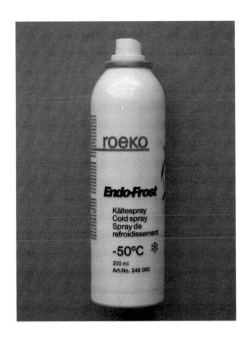

(a)

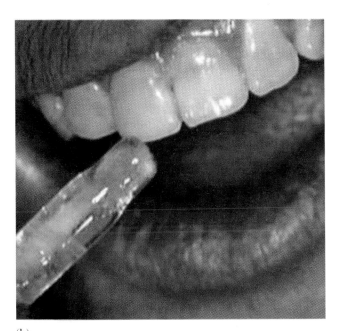

(b)

Fig. A3.18 Cold tests: (a) Endo-Frost® cold spray; (b) an ice stick.

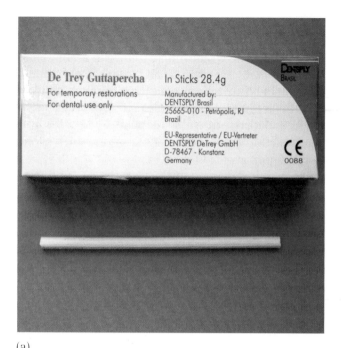

(a)

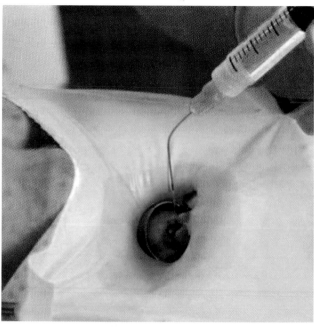

(b)

Fig. A3.19 **(a)** Heat can be applied to an isolated tooth using heated gutta percha sticks. Courtesy of Dr. M. Lessani. (b) Syringed hot water is applied to a tooth isolated with rubber dam.

Radiographic examination

Preoperative periapical radiographs are always taken as part of the diagnostic phase. To gain the most from radiographs they need to be exposed, processed, mounted and labelled correctly. Periapical radiographs are usually the most valuable radiographic views of the teeth and their surrounding periradicular structures. They should be taken using paralleling film holders. This results in undistorted and reproducible images (Fig. A3.20).

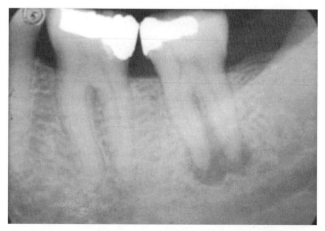

Fig. A3.20 A good diagnostic periapical film showing the tooth under investigation and at least 3 mm of surrounding bone (including a periradicular lesion).

Periapical films may reveal clues about the status of the pulp. There may be obvious signs of pulpal demise, for example, periapical radiolucency or gross caries. However, more subtle signs of pulp status include tertiary dentine, large restorations close to the pulp, pulp calcifications, caries, widening of the periodontal ligament, apical resorption and previous root canal treatment. Periapical films may also reveal signs indicative of a vertical root fracture, that is, visibly separated root fragments, radiolucency along the fracture lines, signs of periodontal-like clinical attachment loss and dislodgment of any root end filling material. It must be remembered that the absence of periradicular radiolucency does not rule out the possibility of a chronic inflammatory process occurring apically. Bone loss as a consequence of an infected root canal system is detected on a radiograph only after there has been significant demineralization of the alveolar bone adjacent to the apices of the affected tooth.

It may be necessary to take additional 'angled' views by changing the horizontal plane of the X-ray tube head by 10–15° in a distal direction to separate otherwise superimposed roots, thus allowing them to be assessed more accurately.

The 'parallax principle' or 'buccal object rule' may be used to locate the relative positions (in the bucco-lingual plane) of two objects to each other, which appear superimposed on one another. The radiographic position of the two objects alters when the angle (either horizontal or vertical) of the X-ray tube and therefore the beam is changed. The more buccal-positioned object will move in the opposite direction to the direction in which the X-ray tube is moved. Lingually/palatally positioned objects will move in the same direction as the change of direction of the X-ray tube (Fig. A3.21(a) and (b)). This is useful when roots overlay each other in the radiographic plane (for example, upper first premolars or to distinguish between the mesial roots of lower first molars).

Bitewing radiographs are a useful adjunct in those cases where the presence of proximal caries needs to be confirmed in relation to the pulp and pulp chamber anatomy. Occlusal radiographs may be used for the radiographic

assessment of trauma to anterior teeth. They are also useful to record lesions that are too large to be viewed on a single standard film (Fig. A3.22).

One of the very few indications for the use of bisecting radiographs is for the detection of possible horizontal root fractures. The fracture lines will only be revealed if the X-ray beam passes within 15° of the plane of the fracture. Therefore, if there is a possibility of a horizontal root fracture, bisecting radiographs should be taken at two or three different horizontal angles in the same vertical plane.

Recently, digital radiography has been introduced in dentistry. Special film sensors (for example, photostimulable phosphor image plates or charged couple devices) that are sensitive to significantly lower doses of radiation from conventional dental X-ray machines are used instead of a conventional X-ray packet. The photostimulable phosphor image plate is placed in a special processor and scanned by a laser, resulting in a digital image. The charged couple device detects the X-ray energy and transfers it to a computer where it is processed into a digital image. The image produced is similar to a conventionally processed X-ray film (Fig. A3.23).

Treatment planning

Once a diagnosis has been reached, the patient should be advised of the various treatment options. For each alternative treatment option, you should advise the patient of the following:

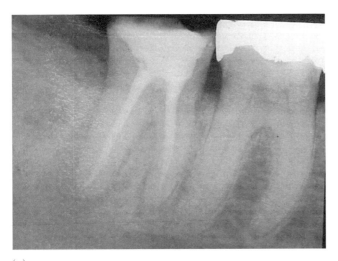

(a)

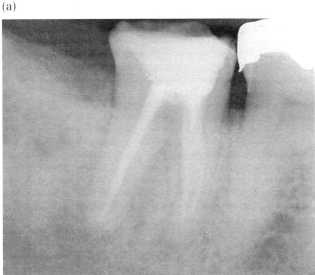

(b)

Fig. A3.21 Parallax views of the mandibular second molar give a better appreciation of the mesial root filling: (a) normal view; (b) distal view.

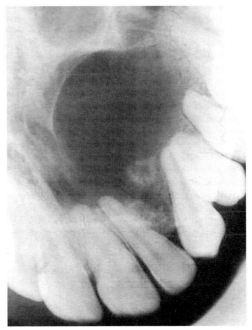

Fig. A3.22 Maxillary occlusal radiographic view of a large periradicular lesion.

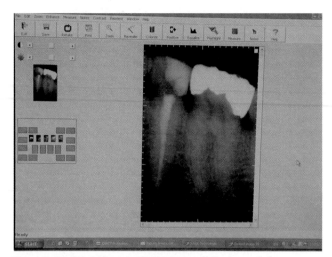

Fig. A3.23 Digital periapical image of the lower left quadrant. Figure courtesy of Dr. S. Rahbaran.

- advantages;

- disadvantages;

- prognosis/likelihood of success of treatment;

- time involved/number of appointments;

- cost implications (when relevant);

- possible complications.

The patient can only make an informed decision on the most suitable treatment once each option has been discussed, but it is your responsibility to advise the patient on the most appropriate treatment option (the principle of informed consent).

What is a treatment plan?

A treatment plan is a list of procedures tailored for each individual patient based on their unique dental problem(s) and needs. The treatment plan aims to address patient care in an ordered, systematic, and logical sequence, and can be broken down into stages:

- pain relief;

- disease stabilization (including oral hygiene instruction, dietary advice, and motivation);

- maintaining/restoring function of teeth;

- maintaining/restoring aesthetics;

- review/maintenance.

A treatment plan may be simple if there is only a solitary problem. In other cases, it may be more complicated, involving a multi-disciplinary approach that needs to be broken down into phases of implementation. The initial treatment plan may have to be modified to allow for

unplanned or unforeseen circumstances. An example of this is where root canal treatment has been planned, but on accessing or removing the existing restoration a vertical fracture line is detected, running mesio-distally (Fig. A3.24). If a fracture such as this runs through the floor of the pulp chamber it could render the tooth untreatable. The treatment plan would obviously need modification as the affected tooth would need extraction (with patient consent) and future treatment options for the resulting space would need to be discussed.

Where does endodontic treatment fit in treatment planning?

Initial phase

The initial phase is for pain relief (for example, pulp extirpation, incision and drainage, or occlusal adjustment).

Definitive phase

The definitive phase is for disease stabilization. The aim is to eliminate dental disease and its aetiological factors (caries stabilization, root canal treatment [including completion of any emergency treatment] and replacement of leaking restorations with well-adapted direct plastic restorations are all stages of disease stabilization). Once root canal treatment has been completed, the tooth should be permanently restored so that it becomes functional again. Root canal treatment may itself improve the appearance of the tooth (e.g. following discolouration due

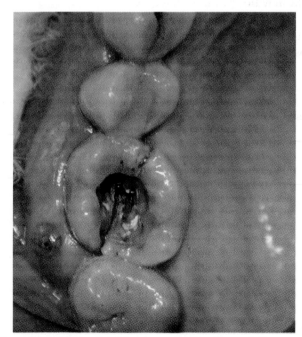

Fig. A3.24 Mesio-distal fracture running through the marginal ridge and cavity of a maxillary molar.

to trauma), but permanent restoration with a veneer or crown (where indicated) may result in a more satisfactory appearance.

Maintenance and review

It is important to assess the outcome of endodontic treatment (see Chapter A7). Review appointments may reveal that treatment has failed and this may mean that retreatment (or revision) is required or the existing treatment plan has to be modified.

Record keeping

It is imperative to record all discussions about treatment options and treatment plans. This provides you with an *aide-mémoire* as treatment progresses and evidence that may be used medico-legally should there be any potential misunderstanding.

What are the factors that influence treatment planning?

Patient factors

The patient's medical history and their history of dental disease and treatment may affect their motivation, attitude to attendance and compliance with treatment. Their expectations must be taken into account as they may be at variance with yours. Occasionally, they may be unrealistic or more importantly, focus on other perceived problems that may not be immediately obvious. One of the great challenges facing you in your practice of dentistry overall is to discern such factors and influence patient behaviour positively.

Dental factors

In terms of dental morphology, endodontic management may be influenced by:

♦ access to the affected tooth;

♦ size of the pulp chamber and presence of calcifications;

♦ number of root canals and their relative size and degree of calcification (Fig. A3.25);

♦ complexity of root canal contour and curvature (Fig. A3.26);

♦ previous root canal treatment and its quality (Fig. A3.27) (presence of foreign bodies, including previous root fillings and separated instruments).

Operator factors

Knowledge, experience and skill are all important in treatment planning. These factors affect the treatment options

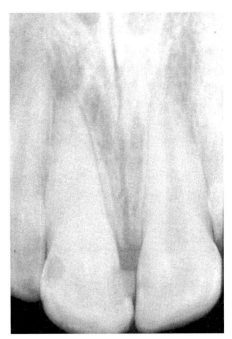

Fig. A3.25 Central incisor with sclerosed pulp chamber and root canal.

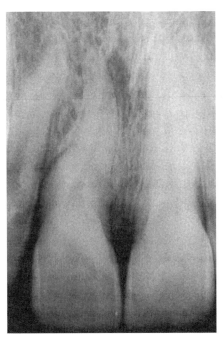

Fig. A3.26 Central incisor with a curved canal system.

offered to the patient and, in due course, the decision-making process. Access to equipment and secondary dental care may also influence the approach adopted.

What does decision making involve?

Decision making involves analysis of all elicited information, prioritizing and 'weighing up' all the pieces of infor-

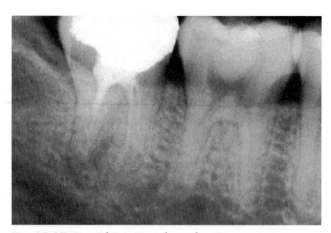

Fig. A3.27 Poor obturation of a molar. Can you improve upon this result?

mation, and giving balanced consideration to the various factors involved. With growing knowledge, confidence and experience, the process of decision making and formulation of treatment plans gradually becomes routine and subconscious. Only when an experienced operator meets an unusual case presentation does the feedback loop break into component parts again. Whilst it can be frustrating to feel slow in the decision-making process as a novice, this step-by-step approach is an essential contributor to the development of competence and, ultimately, expertise.

Preserving pulp vitality

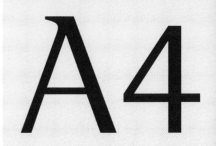

Preserving pulp vitality

Introduction

Any type of active treatment that aims to preserve the health (vitality) of the pulp and prevent potential damage to it is a form of pulp therapy. There are several benefits to preserving pulp vitality (Fig. A4.1). As mentioned previously (in Chapter A2), there are several ways in which the pulp–dentine complex may be breached (or exposed) during restorative treatment.

Attempts at preservation of pulp vitality may be carried out when the pulp is either exposed or very close to being so *only* when following criteria are met:

- the pulp is asymptomatic or has symptoms of reversible pulpitis only;
- there is a normal, positive response to vitality testing;
- radiographic examination reveals no signs of periradicular disease (e.g. widening of the periodontal ligament or periradicular radiolucency).

The outcome of pulp therapy is dependent on:

- removal of noxious stimuli;
- stimulation of a specific dentinogenic response (deposition of sclerotic, reactionary or reparative dentine);
- prevention of future microleakage and future pulp–dentine complex damage.

The actual mode of maintenance of pulp vitality is dependent on the type of exposure (mechanical, carious or traumatic). The most conservative method of pulp preservation should always be attempted first.

- Defensive role (inflammatory response to irritants, secondary and tertiary denture deposition, dentine tubule scleroses)
- Proprioception
- Continued root development in immature teeth

Fig. A4.1 Benefits of preserving pulp vitality.

Procedures to maintain pulp vitality

Stepwise excavation

In situations of potential carious exposure, the amelo-dentinal junction is made caries free. Soft and stained dentine directly overlying the pulp is not excavated to prevent carious exposure; instead, this dentine is dressed *temporarily* with a calcium hydroxide lining and zinc oxide eugenol dressing for at least 8 weeks. The calcium hydroxide lining is placed in direct contact with the carious dentine to:

- eliminate remaining bacteria;
- stimulate remineralization of carious dentine;
- initiate stimulation of reactionary and reparative dentine.

Providing remineralization of the previously soft, demineralized dentine has taken place, the pulp is unlikely to become exposed when the lining and residual caries is excavated (see Chapter B4). It can then be permanently restored. Pulpectomy (root canal treatment) is advisable if a vital pulp response is less certain, the tooth has developed symptoms of pulpitis in the interim, or the pulp becomes exposed during re-excavation.

Indirect pulp capping

This procedure involves leaving soft and carious dentine intentionally over the pulp (caries is cleared from the amelo-dentinal junction), thus preventing exposure. The tooth is then *permanently* restored. The state of the pulp–dentine complex is not re-assessed to confirm whether the carious process in the dentine overlying the pulp has been arrested and becomes, at least, partially remineralized. It must be understood that this treatment may result in undetected carious pulpal involvement, leading to an infected necrotic root canal space requiring subsequent pulpectomy. *We do not recommend this procedure*, but opinion may vary from dental school to dental school.

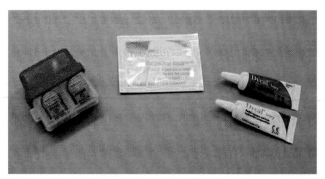

Fig. A4.2 Pulp capping materials (from left to right): dentine bonding resin, Mineral Trioxide Aggregate and calcium hydroxide.

The rationale for both stepwise excavation and indirect pulp capping presumes that the carious dentine immediately overlying the pulp is 'affected' (demineralized) by the overlying carious lesion but not significantly 'infected' by bacteria in caries as the bulk of the infected lesion has been removed. By placing a suitable capping material on this dentine it is thought that the remaining dentine will remineralize.

Direct pulp capping

This involves direct placement of a dressing (pulp capping material) over the mechanically or traumatically exposed pulp. A definitive restoration is then placed over this. A variety of pulp capping materials are currently in vogue (e.g. dentine bonding adhesives, Mineral Trioxide Aggregate and calcium hydroxide) (Fig. A4.2). Until very recently it was thought that all successful capping materials worked by 'gentle' irritation of the underlying pulp tissues causing pulp-derived fibroblasts to differentiate into odontoblasts, which would eventually lay down a dentinal bridge.

Emerging research now suggests that bioactive molecules (e.g. transforming growth factors and bone morphogenetic proteins) are involved in the initiation and regulation of tertiary dentine deposition. Pulp-capping materials are now believed to dissolve components of dentine matrix components, leading to the release of these endogenous bioactive components, the latter stimulating existing odontoblasts to produce reactionary dentine.

Pulpotomy

This involves the surgical removal of inflamed pulp tissue in traumatised teeth, which is excavated until the exposed pulp wound is 'guess-estimated' to be healthy (that is, not inflamed). After pulpotomy has been completed, a dressing is placed over the exposed pulp wound and the tooth is

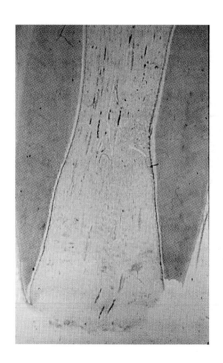

(a)

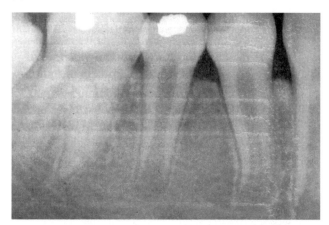

(b)

Fig. A4.3 Immature apices: (a) histological section; (b) radiograph.

restored. This procedure has similar aims as direct pulp capping, however the treatment is clearly more extensive. Pulpotomy has, traditionally, been classified as either a partial ('Cvek') pulpotomy or a coronal pulpotomy and has been historically reserved for application in teeth with immature apices (Fig. A4.3(a) and (b)), hopefully allowing complete root development.

Conclusion

The maintenance of pulp vitality is dependent on a number of factors. If the various dental diseases that can affect the pulp are prevented or adequately treated at

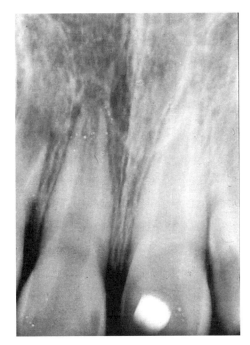

(a)

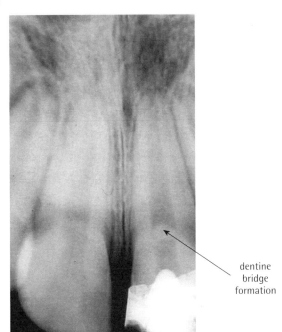

dentine
bridge
formation

(b)

Fig. A4.4 Radiographic evidence of dentine bridge formation in an incompletely formed traumatized tooth: (a) at the time of injury; (b) 1 year later showing continued root development.

an early stage of their development, the pulp–dentine complex will not be significantly affected. It should be remembered, however, that any restorative treatment (for

example, cavity/crown preparation) renders the pulp–dentine complex at risk of damage.

Regular insults to the pulp reduce its recuperative powers and may lead to irreversible effects. Therefore, full consideration should be given to the removal of aetiological factor(s), whilst bearing in mind the possible consequences of the restorative procedures that may lead to further complications as a result of microleakage and the reduced thickness of dentine overlying the pulp. After pulp therapy has been completed, it is imperative to provide an adequate coronal seal. This will prevent contamination of the wound site and subsequent infection, which may go undetected until the status of the pulp has degenerated to an irreversible state.

If haemostasis of the exposed pulp wound cannot be achieved during pulp therapy, then extirpation of the entire pulp may be indicated (pulpectomy). Failure to achieve haemostasis is a sign that the pulp may be irreversibly inflamed or infected, as indeed is very little or no bleeding.

It is always wise to monitor the outcome of the treatment performed on a periodic basis. In addition to checking for any symptoms and signs, the vitality of the tooth should be tested and radiographic examination at 1 year should show signs of formation of a dentinal bridge (Fig. A4.4(a) and (b)). The periodontal ligament should also be intact. The presence of a dentinal bridge (Fig. A4.5) is desirable as it is not only a positive sign of the tooth's vitality, but also serves as a physical barrier to bacterial invasion into the pulp. Interestingly it has been shown that dentinal bridges contain 'tunnel defects', which results in them not being impermeable. It is thought that these deficiencies in the dentinal bridge may be a result of inclusions of blood vessels.

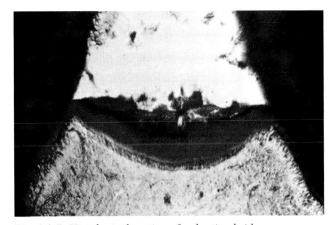

Fig. A4.5 Histological section of a dentine bridge.

Root canal preparation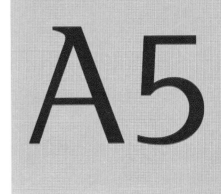

Root canal preparation

What is root canal treatment and why do it?

Root canal treatment can be defined as the removal of inflamed and/or infected pulpal tissue from the root canal system thus *maintaining* periradicular health. In situations where there has been periradicular breakdown (indicated by the presence of a periradicular radiolucent area on a radiograph), root canal treatment will result in the *return to health* of the periradicular tissues. Ultimately, root canal treatment preserves teeth as healthy, functional units within the dental arch.

Root canal treatment is carried out in two phases, which are described as:

+ canal preparation;

+ obturation.

Canal preparation involves the removal of organic material, including pulpal tissue, microorganisms that may have invaded the root canal system and infected dentine from the root canal system. The purpose of obturation is to seal the pulp space to prevent (re-)infection once canal preparation has been completed. Following obturation, provision of a coronal seal and restoration restores the integrity of the tooth. This chapter focuses on the essential elements of preparation; the theory of obturation is covered in the next chapter.

Root canal treatment should always be carried out under rubber dam.

What are the aims of root canal preparation?

The aims of root canal preparation are:

+ the reduction of the bacterial load in the root canal system;

+ the dissolution and debridement of inflamed and infected pulp tissue from the pulp space;

+ creation of a shape suitable for obturation (three-dimensional sealing) of the root canal system.

What does root canal preparation involve?

The preparation of the root canal system involves two elements of activity—these are mechanical and chemical. In reality, the two procedures are carried out simultaneously: *chemo-mechanical* debridement.

Mechanical preparation

A variety of cutting instruments (endodontic files), both hand held and mechanically driven, are used to remove the contents of the pulp space and modify the shape of root canals. The resulting shape should be a *three-dimensionally continuously tapered cone*, widest at the coronal orifice and narrowest at the most apical point of the canal preparation. Ideally, the taper should be centred along the central axis of the original canal and maintain its original contour (Fig. A5.1). The length of the canal being prepared, from

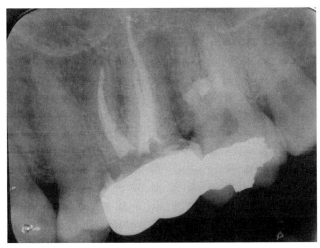

Fig. A5.1 Root filled molar tooth: note the uniform taper of the root canals, and how they follow the root outline.

the occlusal plane or convenient anatomical reference to the most apical point, is termed the 'working length'.

A tapered preparation facilitates:

- improved access for instruments into the root canal to remove infected dentine, pulp tissue and obstructions (e.g. calcifications);

- access for chemical agents (irrigants/medicaments) into the complex root canal system;

- a suitable shape for obturation and three-dimensional sealing.

Chemical preparation

Due to the complex nature of the root canal anatomy (Fig. A5.2(a) and (b)) mechanical instrumentation will not plane the entire root canal surface. Therefore, chemical solutions (irrigants) are used as adjuncts to mechanical preparation. These irrigants prepare the root canal system chemically. Effective irrigants should:

- have an antibacterial action against infected pulpal tissue and dentine;

- flush out pulpal contents and debris created by instrumentation;

- dissolve organic components of pulpal tissue; remnants of organic material can provide substrate for the growth of microorganisms (and their subsequent release of toxic bacterial products into the periradicular tissues—and hence failure of the treatment);

- ease negotiation of canals by acting as a lubricant for instruments;

- help remove the smear layer (a layer of debris that becomes compacted against the canal wall during instrumentation).

The irrigant solution is usually used at concentrations high enough to achieve the above roles without producing irritation to the periradicular tissues. The antibacterial action of chemical irrigation is particularly important in teeth that have become infected.

What are the stages in mechanical preparation?

Mechanical preparation (instrumentation) of the root canal can be divided into the following stages:

- access cavity preparation;
- canal orifice identification;
- coronal flaring and length negotiation;
- apical canal preparation.

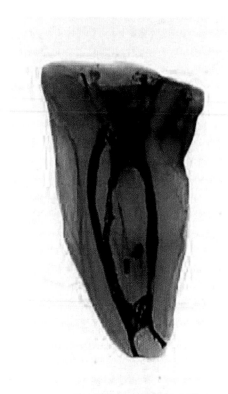

(a)

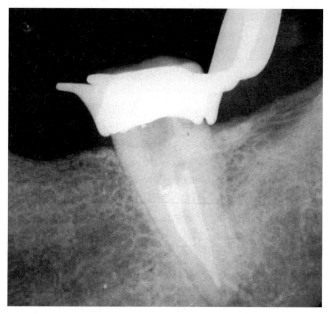

(b)

Fig. A5.2 (a) A cleared mandibular molar tooth with an isthmus between the 2 root canals – irrigant can only reach this area once sufficient access has been created with mechanical instrumentation. (b) An obturated lower mandibular molar tooth – note that the isthmus between the canals has also been sealed.

Maxillary teeth	Root length	Number of canals	Features	Access cavity
				Buccal / Distal — Mesial / Palatal
1	23	1	•Access starting at cingulum and extend towards incisal edge	1 2 3
2	22	1	•Triangular shape to encompass pulp horns •Lateral insisor-apical 3-4 mm has palatal curvature which should always be borne in mind when instrumenting	
3	26	1	•Canine-rounder access cavity then incisors-no need to flare access cavity as there is only 1 pulp horn	
4	21	1=5% 2=90% (B, P) 3=5% (MB,DB, P)	•Initial point of access should be centre of occlusal central groove •Widen access bucco-palatally to locate canal orifices under respective cusp tips (P and B) •Second premolars if only one canal then should be centred and oval in shape (bucco-palatally) to encompass pulp horns •Second premolar canal orifice more centred, if not centred look for second orifice under other cusp tip •Separate canals join apically commonly	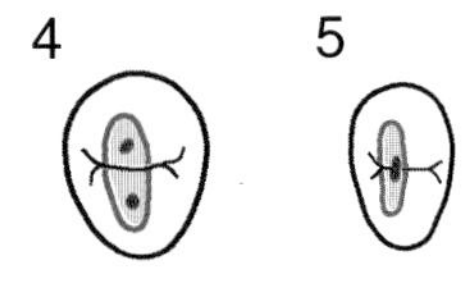 4 5
5	21	1=75% 2=25% (B, P)		
6	22	P longer than MB and DB 3=40% (MB, DB, P) 4=60% (MB1, MB2, DB, P)	•Rhomboid access cavity outline •Distal apect of access cavity is on the mesial aspect of transverse ridge •Palatal canal orifice is usually the largest and therefore easiest to locate •Disto-buccal and palatal orifices usually rounder •Mesio-buccal canal orofice usually more ovoid, reflecting ribbon - shape of the mesio-buccal root •MB2 located between MB1 and palatal canal •Troughing this area with fine burs or ultrasonic tips should eventually reveal an opening of a canal orifice •Lower incidence of MB2 in second molars •DB canal closer to centre of tooth in second and third molars •Increased likelihood of fusion of canals in second and third molars (1 buccal and 1 palatal)	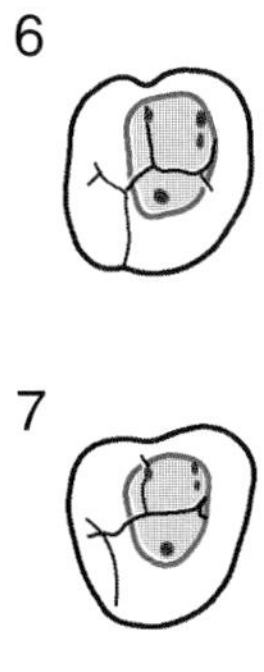 6 7
7	20	P longer than MB and DB 3=60% (MB, DB, P) 4=40% (MB1, MB2, DB, P)		

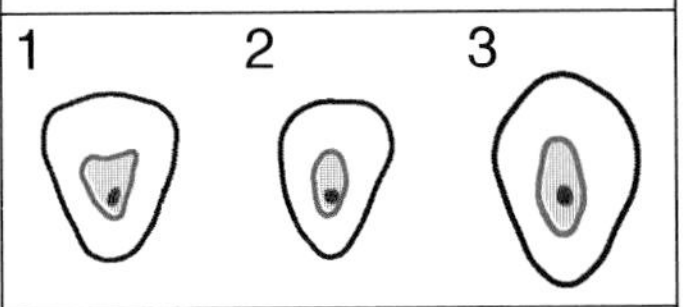

Mandibular teeth	Root length	Number of canals	Features	Access cavity
				Buccal / Distal — Mesial / Lingual
1	21	1=60% 2=40% (B, L)	•Starts at the base of the cingulum •Access cavity should be extended nearly to incisal edge to confirm the presence/absence of the second (lingual) canal	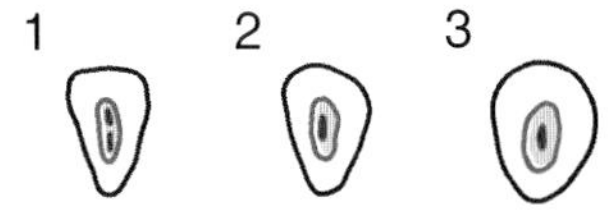 1 2 3
2	21			
3	24	1=90% 2=10% (B, L)	•Starts at the base of the cingulum	
4	22	1=75% 2=25% (B, L)	•Start in central occlusal groove •Access is oval bucco-lingually in shape	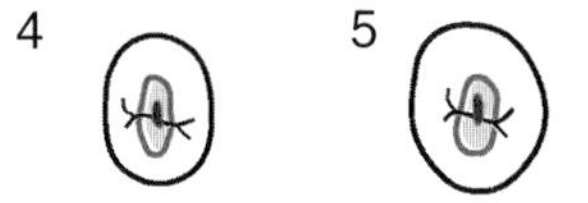 4 5
5	22	1=90% 2=10% (B, L)		
6	21	3=65%(ML, MB, D) 4=35%(ML, MB, DL, DB)	•Mesial canal orifices are found below respective cusp tips •Larger distal canal orifce is more centred •If distal canal orifice is not centred then there is an increased likelihood of a second canal •Increased incidence of fused canals with second and third molars	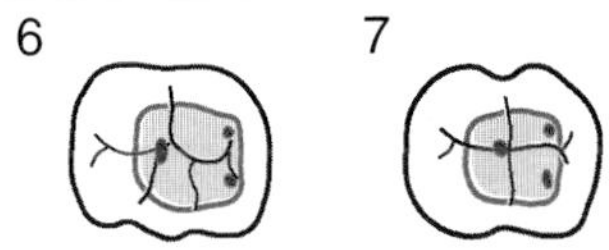 6 7
7	20	3=90% (MB, ML, D) 2=10% (M, D)		

B, buccal; P, palatal; MB, mesio-buccal; DB, disto-buccal; MB1, first mesio-buccal; MB2, second mesio-buccal; L, lingual; ML, mesio-lingual; D, distal; DL, distol-lingual.

Fig. A5.3 Canal features, average lengths and access cavities in various teeth.

Preparation of the root canal system can only be achieved using the correct armamentarium.

Access cavity preparation

The purpose of an access cavity is to remove the roof of the pulp chamber and obtain direct access to the root canal orifices for their subsequent preparation. After accurate diagnosis, the preparation of an access cavity is the first and most important stage of root canal treatment. In order to prepare an adequate access cavity, it is essential to have a basic knowledge of tooth morphology and anatomy, including the number and location of root canals likely to be present in each tooth (Fig. A5.3).

It is common for teeth that require root canal treatment to be heavily restored or carious. Caries and carious restorations must be removed prior to preparing the access cavity in order to prevent infected dentine being introduced inadvertently into the root canal (Fig. A5.4(a)–(c)). Prior to embarking upon root canal treatment, existing restorations should be completely removed if there is any doubt regarding the restorability of the tooth being treated. This allows an objective decision to be made about the viability of the tooth in question. Clearly, the patient must be fully aware of the procedure and have given their consent to exploratory work.

Preparing access cavities in teeth restored with full coverage cast restorations may lead to additional problems:

- The crown may mask the actual orientation of the underlying tooth (for example, being rotated or tilted) thus misleading the operator when attempting to locate the root canal orifices (Fig. A5.5(a);

- Vision may be limited, leading to increased difficulty when locating canal orifices and landmarks that may aid identification. Disorientation can lead to perforations (Fig. A5.5(b–d)).

Caries may be masked radiographically by radiopaque restorations (e.g. metal–ceramic crowns) resulting in an underestimation of the extent of caries involvement. The removal of extracoronal restorations should be considered when:

- caries is extensive and the restorability of the tooth has to be assessed before going ahead with root canal treatment;

- caries excavation or marginal deficiencies result in possible salivary contamination into the pulp chamber (coronal leakage) (Fig. A5.6);

- there is difficulty locating canal orifices;

- a new crown has been planned once the root canal treatment is completed.

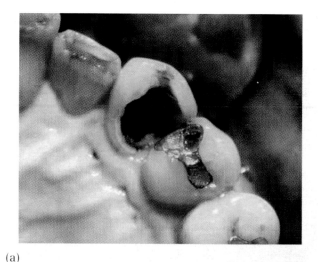

(a)

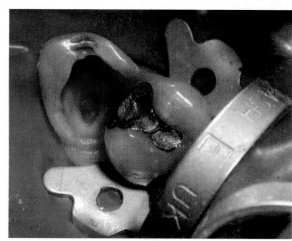

(b)

(c)

Fig. A5.4 (a) A grossly carious and non-vital canine (b) isolated with rubber dam (c) caries excavation prior to commencing root canal treatment. *If there was any doubt regarding the restorability of the tooth the rubber dam would have been placed after caries excavation.*

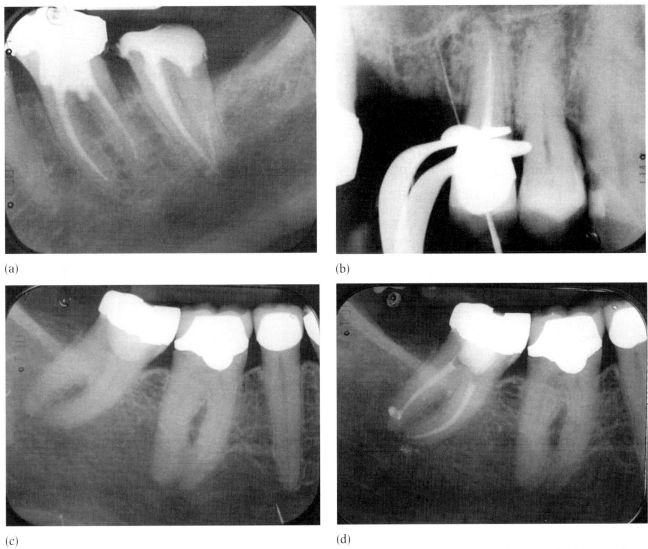

(a) (b)

(c) (d)

Fig. A5.5 (a) Excessive removal of sound dentine from mesial aspect of access cavity and near perforation of pulp cavity floor due to operator losing orientation of the long axis of the tooth (first molar). (b) Perforation due to crown masking natural anatomical landmarks of tooth. (c and d) Radiograph of tilted crowned tooth (second molar) before and after completion of root canal treatment where the operator has followed the long axis of the tooth.

Before starting any treatment on teeth restored with crowns, patients should be advised that they might require a new crown after the root canal treatment has been completed.

The pulp chamber may have to be refined once initial access has been gained to give straight line access to the coronal third of the root canal, which will in turn allow better access for preparation and subsequent obturation (see Fig. B5.7).

Canal orifice identification

The identification and location of root canals can be very time consuming. There is no substitute for having a clean

and disinfected pulp chamber, excellent lighting and magnification. As the roof of the pulp chamber is being removed and the access cavity modified, the cavity should be rinsed regularly with sodium hypochlorite to remove debris and maintain a clear field. This is particularly useful when there is bleeding from pulpal tissue. Viewing the floor of the pulp chamber through irrigant may also provide a small degree of magnification.

Coronal flaring and canal negotiation

Once the orifice of a canal has been located, the root canal should be explored with fine instruments (#08, #10) to

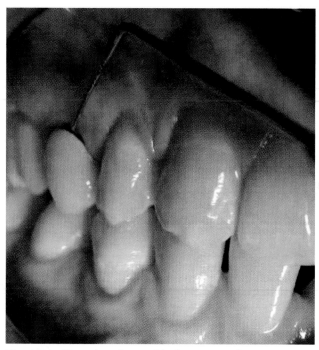

Fig. A5.6 Clinical evidence of leakage around restoration margin.

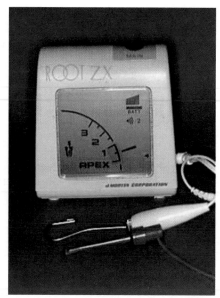

Fig. A5.7 An electronic apex locator (Root ZX apex locator).

ensure it is negotiable. Coronal flaring, the first step in canal preparation, is then performed. It involves the instrumentation of the coronal third to half of the root canal to produce a suitable taper prior to preparation of the apical third of the root canal.

Coronal flaring allows:

- the removal of the bulk of the infected coronal pulp tissue and dentine;

- reduced risk of pushing infected debris/material apically or through to the periradicular tissues;

- the elimination of interferences in the coronal third, thus minimizing the creation of blockages apically;

- early introduction of irrigants into the apical portions of the root canal;

- easier negotiation to the working length;

- improved tactile feedback apically;

- maintenance of the working length during subsequent preparation.

Once the canal has been flared coronally, the full length of the canal should be negotiated and the 'working length' determined. The *working length* starts from the most coronal reference point of the tooth (e.g. cusp/incisal tip), from which measurements may be determined and ends in the apical region of the root canal at a point referred to as the *apical constriction*.

The working length may be estimated by assessing the diagnostic radiographs, but can be measured accurately using an electronic apex locator (Fig. A5.7). This device works by setting up a local electric circuit between the patient's oral mucosa and periodontal ligament at the end of the root canal. It is assumed that the electrical resistance of the periodontal ligament is the same as the oral mucosa. The apex locator consists of a gauge and two terminals. One terminal (shaped like a hook) is attached to the patient's lip and the other terminal clips onto the instrument in the root canal. The gauge registers the resistance between the endodontic file in the root canal

Fig. A5.8 Diagram showing the relationship between the apical constriction, apical foramen and anatomical apex of the root. The apical foramen can be up to 2 mm short of the anatomical apex of the root. The average distance of the apical constriction from the apical foramen is 0.5 mm.

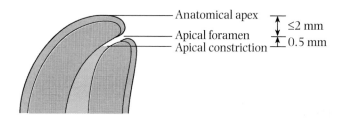

and the oral mucosa. The apex locator's display will indicate when the file makes initial contact ('0' reading) with the periodontal ligament outside the root canal (apical foramen). It is difficult to prepare and obturate up to the apical foramen without potentially extruding excessive material into the periradicular tissues. Therefore, the preparation and subsequent obturation of the root canal should end at the slightly more coronal apical constriction (the narrowest part of the canal). On average, this point lies approximately 0.5 mm short of the apical foramen, therefore once the distance to the apical foramen is known, 0.5 mm can be subtracted to give a working length that should terminate at or very close to the apical constriction (Fig. A5.8).

File	Scanning electron micrograph	Mode of manufacture	Cross-sectional shape	Characteristics	Mode of use
K-Flex file 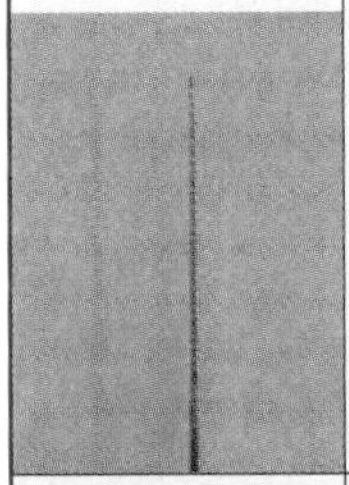	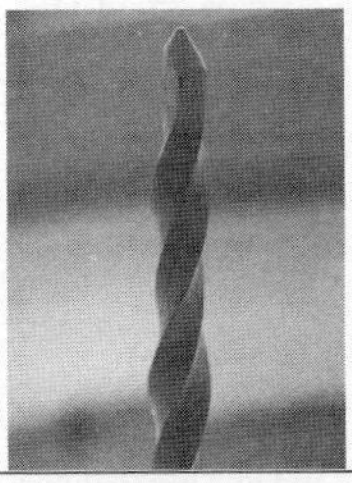	Twisted	Rhomboid	•Good flexibility •Cutting tip •Ideal for negotiating sclerosed canals •Becomes blunt quickly	•Filing •Watch-winding
Flexofile 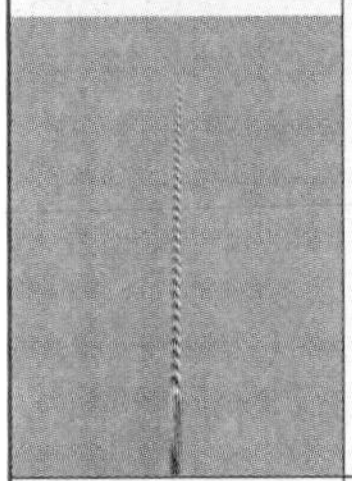	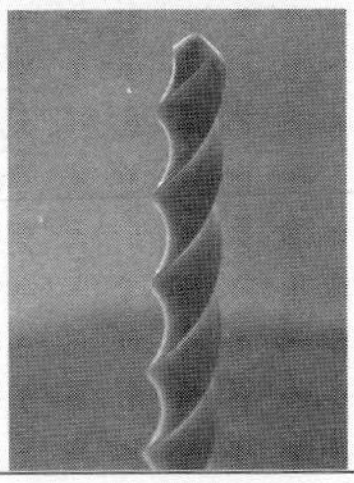	Twisted	Triangle	•Non-cutting tip •Used with 'balanced force technique' •Ideal for preparing curved canals are less likely to gouge dentine	Rotary
Hedstrom 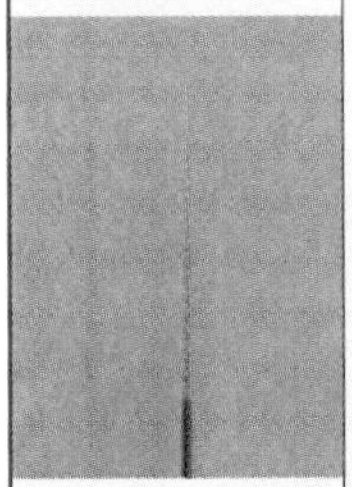	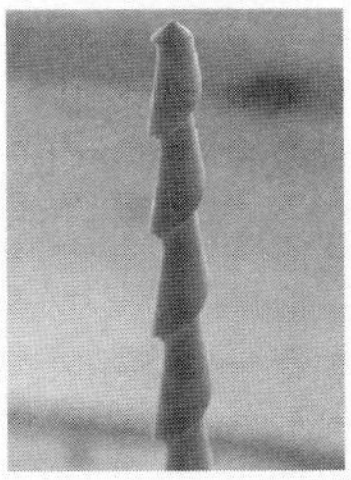	Machined	Round	•Aggressive removal of dentine •Cuts on 'pull' stroke •If rotated more than 30° then increased chance of separation •Ideal for removing gutta percha in re-treatment cases	Filing

Fig. A5.9 Features of different hand files.

Apical canal preparation

After the working length has been determined, the remaining canal may be completely prepared. This is usually carried out in two phases: apical enlargement; and apical taper. The apical third of the canal has to be enlarged to firstly allow adequate penetration and exchange of irrigant and secondly the placement of the subsequent root filling. The manipulation of endodontic files can be divided into a filing motion, rotary motion or a combination of the two.

Historically, the apical portion of the root canal was prepared first, but it became apparent that this style of preparation increased the chances of creating canal aberrations and blockages and was time-consuming to perform. Currently, a coronal-to-apical approach is generally favoured (where the coronal portion of the canal is prepared before the apical portion), regardless of the instruments used.

The technique used to manipulate files in the root canal is determined by a number of factors, which include the following:

The mode of manufacture of the file and its tip design (see Fig. A5.9)

A Hedstrom file, which is made by machining a 'blank' piece of metal alloy, should be used with a filing motion. This type of file will separate (fracture) if rotated more than 30° in either clockwise or anticlockwise directions.

Files that are made by twisting a blank piece of alloy can be used either with a filing motion (for example, K-type files) or with rotary action (for example, Flexofiles) (Fig. A5.9). Files such as Hedstrom have a cutting tip, whereas Flexofiles have a non-cutting tip. The latter design is more likely to result in a smooth-tapered preparation, as the file tip is less likely to gouge the dentine.

Material from which the file is made

Stainless steel files

Small file sizes (06–20) are flexible, but as size increases, flexibility reduces markedly (Fig. A5.10(a) and (b)). This may result in the straightening of curved canals (by uneven removal of dentine from the root canal walls) and in the creation of canal aberrations such as 'zips', 'ledges', 'elbows' and even perforations (Fig. A5.11).

Nickel–Titanium files (Ni–Ti)

Ni–Ti files are super-elastic, which means they retain their flexibility with increased diameter (or taper) when compared to their similar sized stainless steel counterparts (Fig. A5.12(a) and (b)). Many current Ni–Ti instruments are designed for use in a rotary fashion with speed-reducing handpieces, driven by a low-torque electric motor (Fig. A5.13). It may be that you choose to progress to their use in time and with experience. In general, dental schools are moving towards preparation with Ni–Ti files but your school will introduce a reliable method of preparation whether stainless steel or Ni–Ti in design, hand or rotary in operation. A few practical guidelines are provided in Chapter B5.

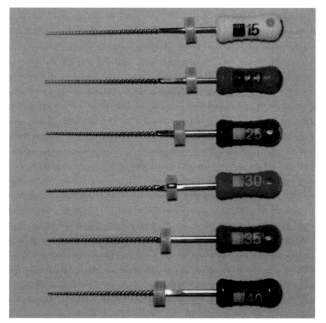

(a)

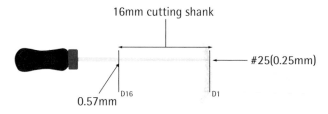

16mm cutting shank

#25(0.25mm)

0.57mm

(b)

Fig. A5.10 (a) Colour-coded Flexofile stainless steel files; note that the rubber stops have been adjusted incrementally so that the operator knows the pre-determined lengths (from #25–40 by 1 mm each) (b) An ISO 0.02 taper size 25 Flexofile. The diameter at the tip of the file (D1) is 0.25 mm, and increases by 0.02 mm per millimetre up the cutting blade of the file (i.e. 0.02 taper). 16 mm from the cutting tip at 'D16' the diameter of the instrument is 0.57 mm (0.32 [0.02 × 16] + 0.25) mm.

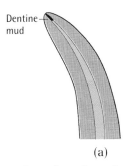

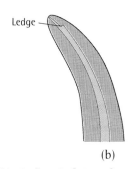

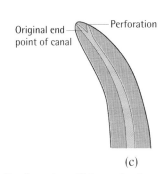

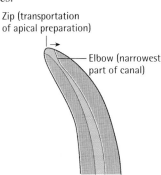

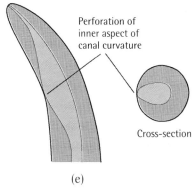

(a) Loss of working length. Loss of working length due to blockage with dentine can be due to: inadequate irrigation, lack of recapitulation, lack of patency filing and over instrumentation with large files.

(b) Ledge. Ledging of curved canals may occur due to: excessive force during instrumentation (especially using files with cutting tips) and failure to pre-curve instruments (K-Flex and Hedstrom files).

(c) Perforation. This can be due to continued filing with large instruments which have not been pre-curved (stainless steel).

(d) Zip and Elbow formation. Hour glass preparation due to large inflexible instruments. Note that the end point of preparation has been 'transported' – the final obturation will be difficult.

(e) Strip perforation. Perforation along the inner curve of the root may occur due to: lack of pre-curving files, aggressive instrumentation (too much force used) and use of large files.

Fig. A5.11 Canal preparation aberrations.

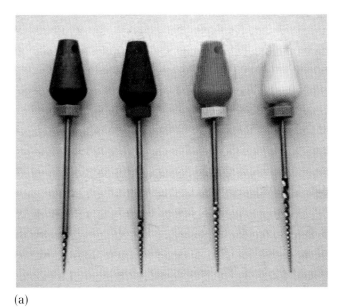

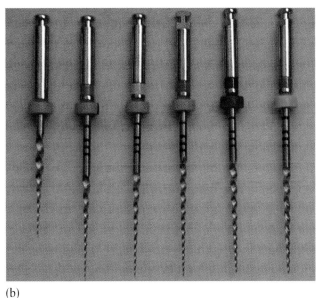

Fig. A5.12 Nickel–Titanium files: (a) Greater Taper® hand files; (b) Protaper® rotary files.

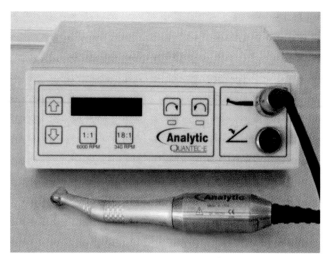

Fig. A5.13 Electric motor with speed-reducing handpiece.

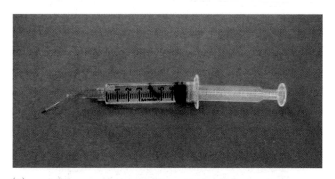

(a)

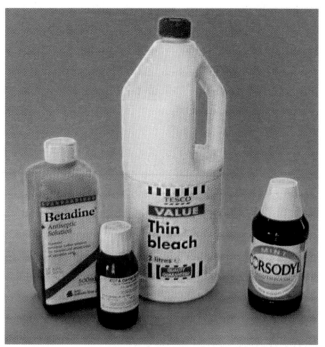

(b)

Fig. A5.14 (a) An endodontic syringe with premeasured needle attached (Monoject®); (b) the tip of the needle has a portion of the tip cut away—this increases the flow of irrigant out of the side of the needle, reducing the chances of extrusion.

The degree of curvature of the canal

There is a greater tendency to create a canal aberration in moderately to severely curved root canals. This is due to an instrument's natural tendency to straighten up (Fig. A5.11). This may be overcome by keeping the apical preparation small when using stainless steel instruments in curved root canals (size 25). The increased flexibility of Ni–Ti instruments means that larger preparations in curved canals may be created with fewer aberrations.

What are the stages in chemical preparation?

Irrigant is usually delivered into the root canal using syringes with fine gauge needles (Fig. A5.14(a) and (b)). A variety of different solutions have been suggested for use as intracanal irrigants, which include sodium hypochlorite, chlorhexidine, iodine-based irrigants, water, saline, hydrogen peroxide and local anaesthetic solution (Fig. A5.15). The greater the volume of irrigant used the more gross debris is flushed out of the canal. However, only an anti-bacterial irrigant will reduce the bacterial load in the root canal system.

The ideal irrigant should be:

◆ antibacterial;

◆ able to dissolve pulpal tissue;

Fig. A5.15 Selection of commonly used irrigants (left to right): Betadine® (iodine-based irrigant), ethylene diamine tetra-acetic acid (E.D.T.A.), bleach (sodium hypochlorite), and Corsodyl® (chlorhexidine).

- cheap;
- easy to use;
- able to have a long shelf life;
- of low surface tension;
- non-staining;
- non-cytotoxic/non-mutagenic;
- compatible with dentine;
- substantive;
- tissue friendly;
- non-toxic;
- non-corrosive to dental equipment/instruments.

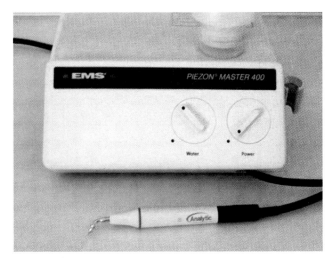

Fig. A5.16 An ultrasonic system.

Sodium hypochlorite

Currently, only sodium hypochlorite fulfils most of these functions. Its antimicrobial properties are due to the action of free chlorine ions, which break down bacterial component proteins into their constituent amino acids, resulting in a significant reduction in the bacterial load in the root canal. A variety of concentrations have been tested and it has been shown that 0.5% is generally as bactericidal as 5%. However, the more concentrated the sodium hypochlorite, the greater its tissue-dissolving power, a function that may also be increased by warming the solution. To optimize the benefits of sodium hypochlorite, it is advisable to replenish the bleach in the root canal as the irrigant becomes depleted of its free chlorine ions. The bleach should also be gently agitated to circulate the irrigant into the inaccessible areas of the root canal system during instrumentation.

Other irrigants

Microorganisms found in retreatment cases (for example, *Enterococcus faecalis*) may be more resistant to the effects of sodium hypochlorite. It has been suggested that alternating irrigation of sodium hypochlorite with iodine-based irrigants (for example, iodine potassium iodide) may be more effective in their elimination. Chlorhexidine solutions (for example, Corsodyl®) have also been suggested for use in retreatment cases. Both alternatives are antibacterial, but their major disadvantage when compared to sodium hypochlorite is that they are not able to dissolve organic pulp tissue.

Ultrasonic instrumentation

Files may be made to vibrate at very high frequencies by generating acoustic energy (2–30 kHz), which can be transmitted to the file as mechanical energy. Initially, these

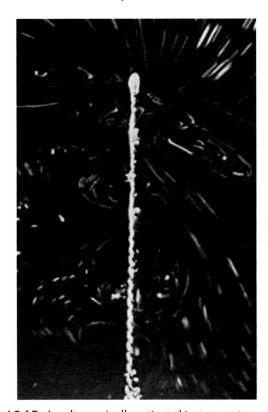

Fig. A5.17 An ultrasonically activated instrument.

files were introduced for purposes of canal preparation, but due to the increased incidence of canal aberrations their role is now advocated as an 'energizer' of irrigant and to aid flushing the root canal once preparation has been completed (Fig. A5.16).

When files are ultrasonically activated in the root canal the irrigant immediately surrounding the file becomes turbulent (acoustic streaming), resulting in the irrigant penetrating the more inaccessible areas of the root canal system (Fig. A5.17). In order for acoustic streaming to take place, the canal has to be wide enough to allow the activated file to have unrestrained movement, otherwise it will become dampened against the canal wall and may lead to the creation of aberrations. Ultrasonic irrigation should therefore only be attempted after the canal has been prepared completely. For example, an activated size 15 ultrasonic file will only be effective in a canal that has been prepared for a file up to size 40.

What is the smear layer and what is its relevance to endodontic treatment?

The smear layer is an amorphous film of organic and inorganic material generated from instruments contacting the root canal walls. It has been described as 'bi-laminar' in structure as it is composed of a superficial layer on the root canal surface (1–2 μm) and plugs penetrating up to 40 μm into the dentinal tubules (see Fig. A2.19).

Its thickness and composition are related to a number of factors, which include design of instrument(s) used, preparation technique, forces used during mechanical preparation, and also the choice of irrigant and possibly how it was activated (e.g. with ultrasonic files).

Suggested advantages for the retention of the smear layer are that its presence may:

* slow down bacterial invasion;
* block tubules which, in its absence, would be difficult to access and clean;
* have an inhibitory affect on bacterial growth.

However, removal of the smear layer may also be beneficial in that:

* it harbours bacteria and may also act as nutriment for bacteria;
* it may act as a barrier to irrigant and medicament penetration;
* if and when it disintegrates, it will affect the seal of the root canal obturation material;
* it may influence the quality of the bond obtainable with sealers.

What is the purpose of intracanal medication?

The elimination of bacteria from the root canal is difficult to achieve with chemo-mechanical instrumentation alone. Therefore, to reduce the bacterial load further, placement of an antibacterial medicament in the root canal between the preparation and obturation phase is advisable (that is, a multi-visit strategy—see Chapter B5).

The functions of an ideal intracanal medicament are to:

* further reduce bacterial load;
* provide a 'secondary' barrier against coronal leakage between visits.

Leaving the root canal empty between appointments or with an inappropriate intracanal dressing (that is, not adequately antibacterial) is not advisable because the small number of surviving microorganisms in the root canal will proliferate rapidly, resulting in the bacterial load returning back to its initial levels within days after chemo-mechanical preparation.

As well as eliminating bacteria, certain medicaments have other desirable properties including:

* aiding in the dissolution of necrotic pulpal tissue by its synergistic effect with sodium hypochlorite used at subsequent visit(s);
* helping to dry persistently weeping canals;
* a sedative effect (for example, Ledermix®) (Fig. A5.18) on irreversibly inflamed vital pulps that have not been completely extirpated (see below).

The two commonly used intracanal medicaments are calcium hydroxide and Ledermix®, although recently it has been suggested that chlorhexidine gel may also be used.

Calcium hydroxide

Calcium hydroxide is usually the intracanal medicament of choice (Fig. A5.19(a) and (b)). Not only is it an effective bacteriostatic dressing, it is also able to hydrolyse pathogenic components of bacteria such as the lipopolysaccarides. This dressing is available as a powder, which is mixed with sterile distilled water into a paste. Various

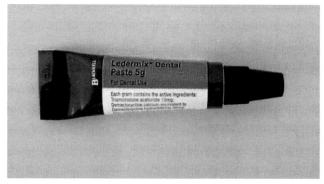

Fig. A5.18 Ledermix® paste.

manufacturers produce ready-mixed dressings available in cartridge form, which may be applied directly into the root canal. There is evidence to suggest that a minimum dressing time with calcium hydroxide of at least 1 week will significantly reduce the bacterial load in teeth with infected root canals compared to either leaving the root

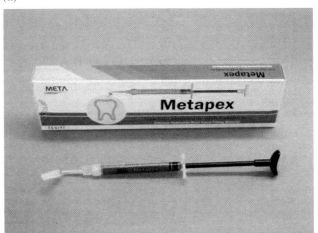

(a)

(b)

Fig. A5.19 (a) Calcium hydroxide comes as a powder, which has to be mixed with sterile water (top), or in ready-prepared syringes (middle and bottom); (b) Metapex®—calcium hydroxide and iodine mixture in a preprepared syringe (suggested for re-treatments, as it may be more effective against the different type of flora found in these cases).

canals empty or dressing with other medicaments. Calcium hydroxide is also effective in canals that persistently weep tissue fluid.

Ledermix®

Ledermix® is a paste containing a steroid (triamcinalone) and an antibiotic (demeclocycline [tetracycline]). This dressing may be used in cases where the pulp is acutely inflamed and requires immediate treatment but adequate anaesthesia is unobtainable, preventing complete pulp extirpation. If there is inadequate time to extirpate a pulp completely, Ledermix® may be used as an intracanal medicament to relieve symptoms in the short term. It must be recognized that this is, in effect, a 'quick fix' and is *not* an alternative to effective treatment (that is, total extirpation). It is also fundamental to realize that Ledermix® can only be effective on vital pulp tissue and therefore it has no place as an intracanal medicament in non-vital cases or in cases where root canal preparation has been completed.

Why is a good temporary restoration important?

Before removing the rubber dam and discharging the patient, it is essential that a good quality temporary restoration is placed in the access cavity to prevent re-contamination of the root canal.

Intermediate restorative material (IRM) (Fig. A5.20) or glass ionomer cement (Fig. A5.21) are ideal interim

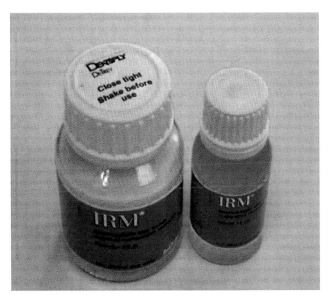

Fig. A5.20 Intermediate restorative material.

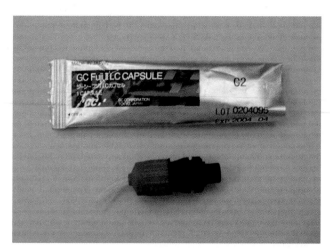

Fig. A5.21 Glass ionomer (Fuji LC) cement.

restorations. Failure to provide an adequate coronal seal even at this stage will result in the disinfected root canals becoming infected with microorganisms from the saliva and in some cases these microorganisms may be more virulent and subsequently extremely difficult to eliminate.

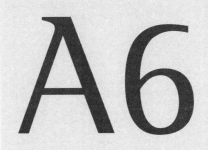

Obturation of root canals

Obturation of root canals

Why is it necessary to obturate root canals?

Current preparation techniques do not eliminate microorganisms completely, therefore root canal obturation is necessary in order to:

- entomb any remaining microorganisms within the root canal system;
- prevent re-infection by denying new microorganisms (within saliva) entrance into the tooth;
- prevent entry of periradicular tissue fluid which may be a continuing nutritional supply for the remaining microorganisms, inhabiting the root canal system (Fig. A6.1).

When should canals be obturated?

Root canals should be obturated only when they have been completely prepared. The ideal time to obturate is when there are fewest microorganisms in the system. This is why it is argued that every effort should be made to complete root canal treatment of cases with inflamed vital (non-infected) pulps at the same visit as root canal preparation, because the risk of coronal leakage through temporary restorations between appointments may result in infection of the root canal (see 'Single- and multiple-visit root canal treatment').

Historically, infected teeth were subjected to microbiological sampling techniques to identify the presence of microorganisms. When the results were negative it was deemed the appropriate time to obturate. Unfortunately, the tests performed were time consuming and impracticable. In the absence of reliable bacterial sampling protocols, it is imperative that adequate chemo-mechanical preparation techniques be performed under aseptic conditions and, where appropriate, the root canals may be dressed with an interappointment intracanal medication.

Fig. A6.1 Root-filled maxillary molar—a good quality root filling should three-dimensionally seal the root canal space without any voids.

Single- and multiple-visit root canal treatment

In situations where the tooth undergoing root canal treatment is vital (for example, following carious exposure or where there are symptoms of irreversible pulpitis), once the canal system has been completely prepared it may be obturated at the same visit (single-visit root canal treatment) if there is sufficient time. Root canal systems that are infected (i.e. showing signs of periradicular periodontitis) are more challenging to disinfect adequately due to their increased bacterial load. Therefore, once preparation has been completed the canals should be dressed with an antibacterial inter-appointment dressing (for example, non-setting calcium hydroxide) for at least 7 days to further reduce the bacterial load before obturation.

It is generally agreed that there are some cases that need to be addressed by a multiple-visit treatment strategy. These include:

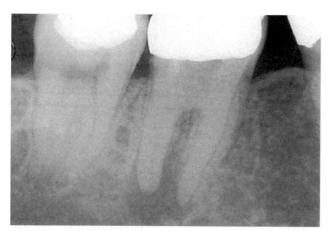

Fig. A6.2 Mandibular molar with asymptomatic periradicular lesion.

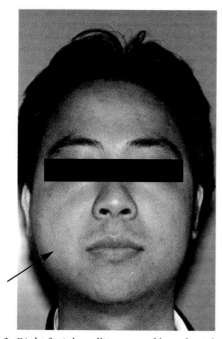

Fig. A6.3 Right facial swelling caused by a dental abscess.

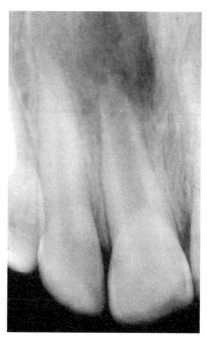

Fig. A6.4 Periapical radiograph showing incomplete root development on an upper central incisor.

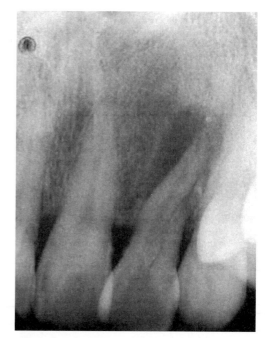

Fig. A6.5 Radiograph of tooth with complex root canal anatomy.

- non-vital teeth with a symptomless periradicular lesion (Fig. A6.2);
- weeping/wet canals that cannot be dried successfully;
- acute infections/abscesses (Fig. A6.3);
- large open apices (Fig. A6.4);
- difficult anatomy requiring a lengthy preparation time to allow adequate time for irrigant to be effective (Fig. A6.5);
- revision of pre-existing, failing root canal treatment (Fig. A6.6).

When multiple-visit root canal treatment is being carried out, obturation should only be considered when:

- canals can be dried easily;
- patient's symptoms and signs have improved;
- no swelling is present.

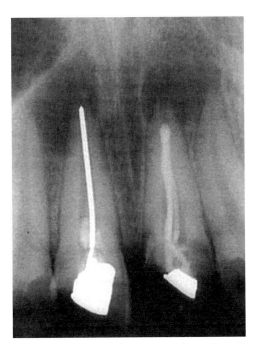

Fig. A6.6 Radiograph revealing poor technical quality of root canal treatment with obvious periradicular disease. Note the 'empty' space between the single root filling points and the root canal walls.

What materials are used for obturation?

At present gutta percha is the most suitable material to predictably and simply obturate the root canal system. The ideal root filling material should:

- be biocompatible;
- be bactericidal/bacteristatic;
- be radiopaque;
- be easy to introduce into the root canal;
- have a long working time;
- be dimensionally stable and impervious to fluids;
- be sterile;
- have a long shelf life;
- be cheap;
- be safe to use;
- be easily removed;
- be non-toxic;
- be non-mutagenic and non-carcinogenic.

Gutta percha

The most commonly used obturation material is gutta percha (GP) (Fig. A6.7). It remains the root filling material of choice, as it closely resembles the properties of an ideal root filling. It is composed of zinc oxide (60–75%), GP (19–22%), opacifiers (barium sulphate (1–17%)), waxes and resins (1–4%)). Gutta percha is a polymer derived from the taban tree and is an isomer of rubber. It can be used at room temperature and with heat or softening agents (for example, chloroform).

It is used in conjunction with a sealer to produce a homogeneous mass to seal the root canal space. Gutta percha is manufactured in standard International

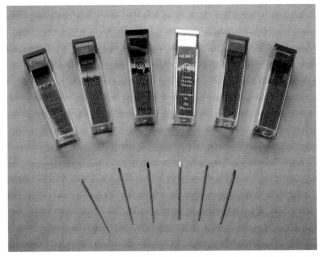

Fig. A6.7 Gutta percha points of various sizes being used to obturate a central incisor.

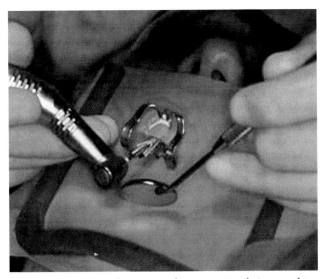

Fig. A6.8 International Standards Organization (ISO) sized gutta percha points, sizes 30–55 (left to right) and 0.02 mm taper. Courtesy of Dr. M. Lessani.

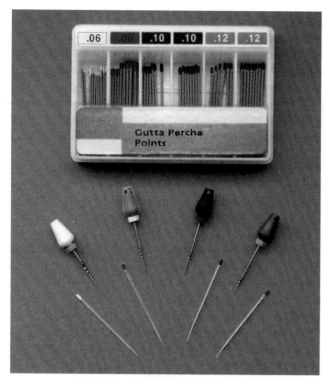

Fig. A6.9 Non-standardized Greater Taper® gutta percha points with the same tip diameter (#20) and taper (left to right 0.06, 0.08, 0.10, 0.12 mm) as the Greater Taper® files. In theory, when canals are prepared to a predetermined taper using these Nickel–Titanium files, the corresponding size Greater Taper® gutta percha point should fit the prepared canal.

Standards Organization sizes of 0.02 mm taper (Fig. A6.8) and non-standardized sizes of various tapers and sizes (Fig. A6.9).

Sealers

The main function of sealers is to fill in the voids between the root canal wall and the GP root filling and also between individual GP points (when lateral condensation is being used). Sealers should be used sparingly. Several 'families' of sealer are available. These include zinc oxide-based sealers, [Kerr's Tubliseal® (Fig. A6.10) and Roth's® sealer (Fig. A6.11)], calcium hydroxide-based sealers, for example, Sealapex® (Fig. A6.12), and resin-based sealers (for example, AH plus® (Fig. A6.13)). The zinc oxide-based variety has the longest track record and is favoured by the authors. Your dental school will introduce you to one or two examples.

Other materials

Historically, formaldehyde (mummifying) agents and rigid cores (silver points (Fig. A6.14(a), (b) and (c)) and acrylic

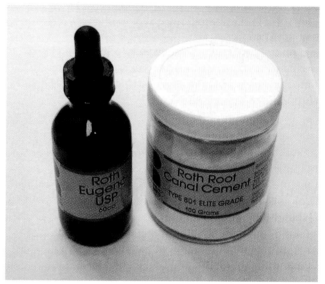

Fig. A6.11 Roth's® sealer.

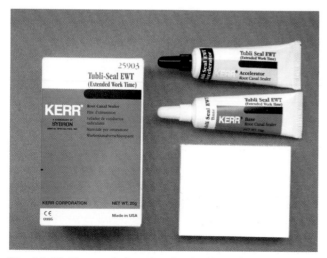

Fig. A6.10 Zinc oxide-based sealer (Tubliseal®). Courtesy of Dr. M. Lessani.

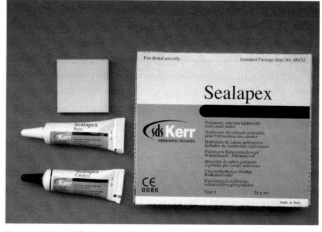

Fig. A6.12 Calcium hydroxide-based sealer (Sealapex®). Courtesy of Dr. M. Lessani.

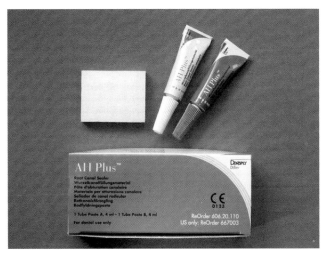

Fig. A6.13 AH plus® resin sealer. Courtesy of Dr. M. Lessani.

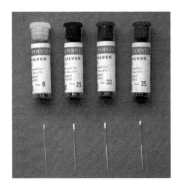

(a)

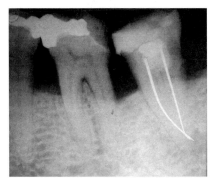

(b)

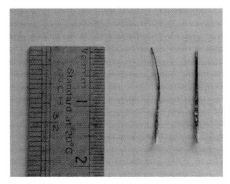

(c)

Fig. A6.14 (a) Silver points; (b) failing silver point root filling (note the periradicular radiolucency); (c) silver points removed after re-root canal treatment – note that the silver points are black due to corrosion.

points) were used to seal root canals. Formaldehyde pastes (for example, N_2-endomethasone) have been shown to cause severe and sometimes irreversible damage when extruded into the periradicular tissues (for example, tissue necrosis and paraesthesia). The use of rigid silver points was popular during a period where root canal treatment was accepted to be difficult to carry out. They were easily introduced into root canals and were stiff enough to reach the working length, but did not result in three-dimensional obuturation of the root canal space.

What is the ideal level of obturation?

The obturation material should extend through the full length of the root canal, from the canal orifice to the apical constriction (Fig. A6.15). There are several obturation techniques currently in vogue and they all aim to produce a dense, homogeneous, three-dimensionally filled root canal system. The use of cold obturation techniques should ensure control, in particular of the length of the root filling (see Chapter B6). The obturation material should reach a predetermined length and be adapted well to the surrounding area. The apical portion (apical 3 mm) should be composed more of the core-obturating material (that is, GP) than sealer.

Selection of the master GP point is a crucial step in obturation. The master point should fit snugly in the apical portion of the root canal. The term 'tug-back' has been used to describe the tight feeling the GP gives when tried in. It is assumed that this tug-back is always at the full working length but it may in fact be due to the complexities of the root canal system and curvatures in planes not shown on the radiographs.

Care should be taken to avoid the use of small GP points, which may go beyond the working length and if forced into the periradicular tissues may induce an inflammatory or foreign body reaction.

Cold lateral condensation versus thermoplasticized techniques

The use of heat results in a more homogenized mass of GP. This may create a root filling that is closer to the 'ideal' as

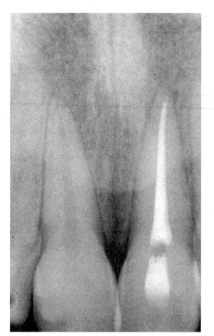

Fig. A6.15 Radiograph of a well-condensed and extended root filling, terminating at the apical constriction.

it is more dense and contains less voids, yet the cold lateral condensation technique is still very widely used and taught. Lateral condensation is relatively easy to learn and can result in the production of well-adapted root fillings. Its results are predictable if carried out correctly and it is still the standard against which other techniques are compared in research studies. Chapter B6 describes the technique.

Coronal seal

The long-term success of any root canal treatment depends on ensuring that microorganisms are prevented from re-entering the root canal system after obturation (Fig. A6.16(a)–(c)). Chapter B6 describes various techniques of coronal restoration, depending upon the individual tooth in question.

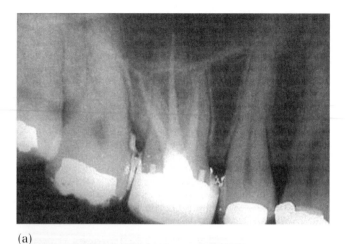

(a)

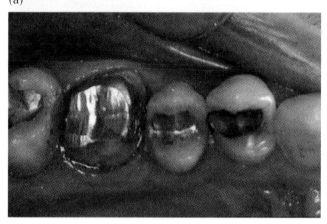

(b)

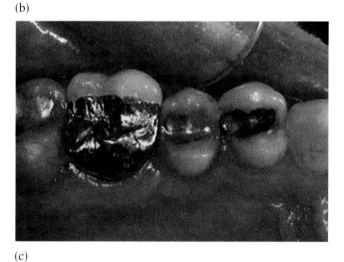

(c)

Fig. A6.16 (a) Radiograph of root filled molar; (b) coronal core preparation; (c) extracoronal metal-ceramic restoration.

Treatment outcomes

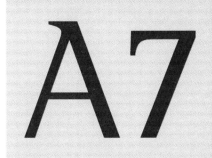

Treatment outcomes

What is successful root canal treatment?

The ultimate aim of root canal treatment is to maintain teeth as healthy functional units by either preventing periradicular periodontitis or, where periradicular periodontitis is already present, creating an environment conducive to healing.

After completion of root canal treatment, a note should be made of the patient's symptoms and signs and these should be compared with the symptoms and signs prior to treatment. Successful elimination of the causal factors of inflammatory breakdown in the pulpal or periradicular tissues should result in the presentation of no new symptoms, and the resolution of any existing symptoms and signs.

The patient's perception of success after treatment is subjective and may differ from that of the clinician, who is trained to develop a critical and objective analysis of the outcome of treatment. Patients may well regard the retention of an asymptomatic, but functional, root-filled tooth as a successful outcome whereas clinical examination may reveal clear signs of lack of success (Fig. A7.1(a) and (b)). Examination may even indicate features that point to failure of treatment, for example, tenderness to palpation, presence of a sinus tract, or development, increasing size or no improvement in size of existing periradicular radiolucencies (refer, for example, to Fig. B7.6(a) and (b)). This two-stage assessment, although essential, may therefore provide confusing information, relying as it does on the patient's reported symptoms on the one hand and the clinical findings on the other.

The absence of any symptoms should not be relied upon, in isolation, to assess the outcome of treatment. There will be situations (for example, chronic periradicular periodontitis) where the treated tooth has never been symptomatic, but radiographic examination reveals the presence of periradicular radiolucency. The absence of symptoms does not provide clear evidence of healing. Further, it is not uncommon for symptoms to improve slowly over several months (for example, patients who have had long-standing chronic pain prior to treatment). In this situation, the patient may only report a slight improvement or may not even be entirely sure if there has been any improvement in the symptoms at all. There are also occasions when patients are unsure of the outcomes of treatment, particularly when the clinician attempts to elicit signs of improvement.

A radiograph at the time of the re-assessment appointment serves as a useful and sometimes more objective

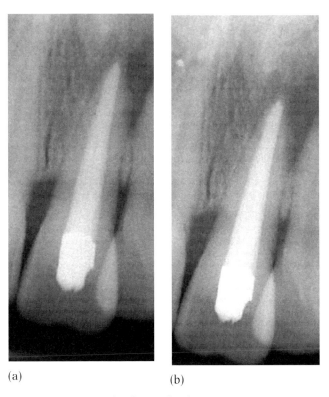

(a)   (b)

Fig. A7.1 Sequential radiographs showing no improvement in size of periradicular lesion following root canal treatment (a) and 1 year later (b). The adjacent teeth respond positively to vitality testing.

method of evaluating the outcome of treatment than the clinical examination, in particular in assessing if there has been any periradicular tissue regeneration or breakdown.

After gaining as much information as possible from the clinical and radiographic examination, the next stage is to assimilate this information and determine if the treatment carried out has, in fact, resulted in a successful outcome. The outcome of endodontic treatment may be broadly grouped into three categories: successful healing, uncertain healing or failure to heal. Treatment can only be regarded as a success when certain criteria are met. These criteria relate to:

+ the patient's reported symptoms;
+ the clinical signs;
+ radiographic findings.

The probability of achieving a successful outcome is increased when the following have been achieved:

+ correct initial diagnosis;
+ disinfection of as much of the root canal space as possible;
+ three-dimensional sealing of the disinfected root canal space;
+ immediate placement of a permanent coronal seal over the root canal space to prevent infection/re-infection.

What influences the outcome of root canal treatment?

Several studies have been published attempting to assess the factors that may influence the outcome of endodontic treatment. However, due to their heterogeneity, only a limited number of factors have been shown to have a strong influence on the prognosis of treatment. In essence, all causes of failure are ultimately attributable to residual infection and re-infection of the root canal space with microorganisms,

Observable factors affecting outcome

The following observable factors affect outcome:

+ pre-operative status of the tooth (presence/absence of a periradicular area);
+ level of obturation (Fig. A7.2(a) and (b));
+ quality of obturation (including lateral seal) (Fig. A7.3);
+ coronal leakage (Fig. A7.4);
+ whether the treatment performed was a revision of an existing root canal treatment (retreatment).

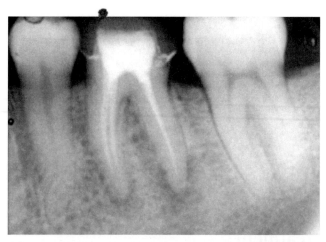

(a)

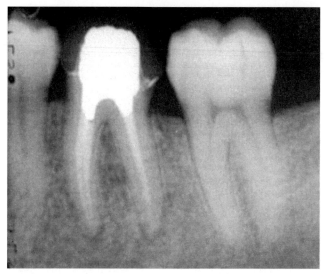

(b)

Fig. A7.2 (a) Short and underprepared root canal fillings in this molar with periradicular radiolucencies. A radiograph taken following retreatment (b) suggests that healing is now proceeding. Note the wider preparation and that the root filling (and therefore the preparation) have been extended to the correct working length.

Factors that have a primary influence on outcome

Pre-operative status of tooth

Teeth that are vital or have an infected necrotic pulp space with no evidence of periradicular breakdown (i.e. an intact lamina dura and periodontal ligament) should have a success rate in the region of 95%. This is a 10–15% higher success rate than those cases with radiographic signs of chronic periradicular periodontitis before treatment begins. This is due to the significantly higher bacterial load in the root canal space of teeth with signs of

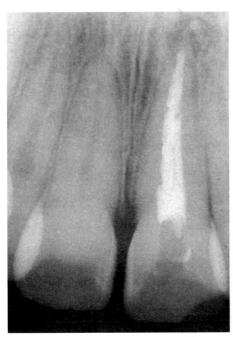

Fig. A7.3 Although this root filling is of adequate length, the numerous voids are a sign that the root treatment is not of a satisfactory standard. This has resulted in the patient complaining of persistent pain, and also explains the presence of the periradicular radiolucency.

periradicular periodontitis (which is more difficult to reduce below the desired threshold for healing to occur).

From the evidence available, it appears that modern treatment techniques and protocols still have room for

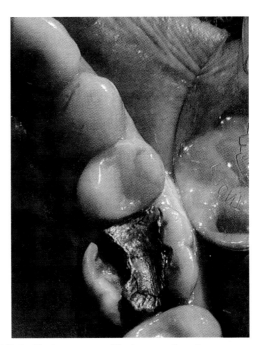

Fig. A7.4 Obvious coronal leakage and caries.

improvement. They certainly appear to be unable to consistently reduce the higher bacterial load in teeth with chronic periradicular periodontitis to the same levels as teeth without these signs.

Apical level to which the root canal space is sealed

Root canal preparation and sealing of the root canal should terminate at the apical constriction (usually within

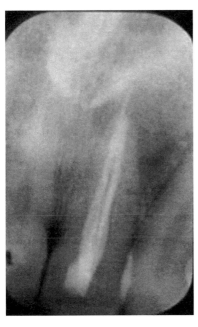

(a)

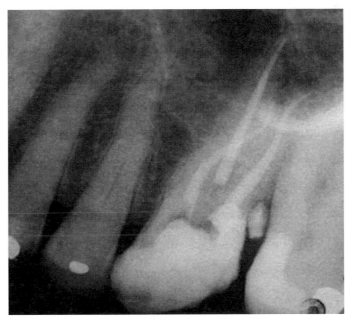

(b)

Fig. A7.5 (a) An overextended and inadequately obturated root canal; (b) over extended root filling in the palatal root.

2 mm of the radiographic apex). Overfills into the surrounding periradicular tissues (Fig. A7.5) and root fillings that appear to be more than 2 mm short of the radiographic apex result in a higher rate of failure. Overextended root fillings are usually relatively well tolerated by the periradicular tissues; it is the overpreparation that precedes a 'long' root filling (i.e. unintentional instrumentation into the periradicular tissues) that could result in the extrusion of microorganisms into the periradicular tissues. Inability to eliminate such microorganisms may lead to treatment failure. Root canal spaces that are sealed well short of the radiographic apex may not have been totally prepared, therefore leaving residual infection, which may remain in the unsealed portion of the root canal space (Fig. A7.6).

Quality of obturation

Voids in a root filling (Figs. A7.3 and A7.5a) indicate empty spaces within the root canal which may allow tissue fluid to percolate into the canal and become a source of nutrition for bacteria that may still be present within the tooth. A poorly sealed root filling will also mean that if coronal leakage occurs, bacteria are more likely to cause periradicular breakdown as they may proliferate relatively easily within the empty spaces between the root filling and root canal walls.

Coronal leakage

After completion of root canal treatment, a well-adapted coronal seal is required to prevent contamination of the

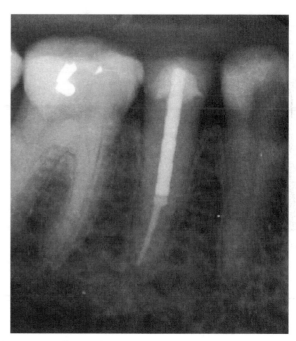

Fig. A7.7 Radiograph of a post-retained crown. Note that below the post, at least 5 mm of apical gutta percha has been left undisturbed.

sealed, disinfected root canal space. Evidence is steadily emerging that the lack of a good coronal seal increases the potential for re-infection and adversely affects the outcome of root canal treatment. Teeth that are restored with post-retained restorations should have at least 4–5 mm of intact root filling apical to the intraradicular post. The failure rate increases when there is less than 5 mm of root filling remaining apically (Fig. A7.7).

Root canal re–treatment

Cases that are re-treated (revised) due to signs of failure (i.e. chronic periradicular periodontitis) have been reported to have a success rate in the region of 70%. This may be due to the presence of obstructions (for example, the inability to completely retrieve previous root filling material and canal aberrations [ledges and blockages]) preventing the desired working length from being reached (Fig. A7.8a and b). This will result in certain areas of the root canal space being inadequately disinfected or sealed. The situation may also be compounded by the fact that the microbial flora in re-treatment cases may be persistent and particularly virulent (for example, due to the presence of *Enterococcus faecalis*).

Endodontically treated cases that appear successful clinically and radiographically but are inadequate technically should be re-treated prior to provision of cast restorations, as the poor technical appearance of a root filling is generally indicative of poor disinfection. In these situations the

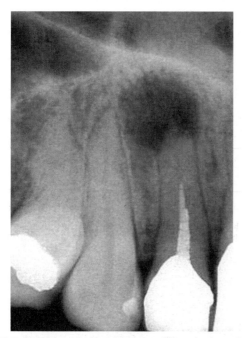

Fig. A7.6 Radiograph of a short root filling with visible patent root canal space apically and evidence of periradicular disease.

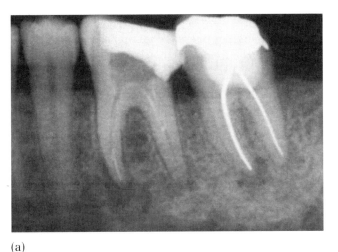
(a)

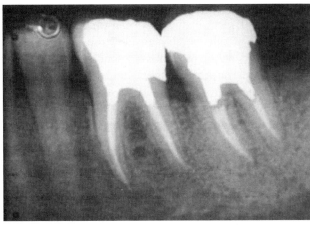
(b)

Fig. A7.8 (a) These root-treated teeth are failing (chronic periradicular periodontitis). Failure is probably due to a combination of inadequate root canal preparation and obturation (lower first and second molar teeth) and a lack of an adequate coronal seal (lower left first molar). (b) Both teeth have been re-root treated—note that the separated instrument in the mesio-buccal canal of the first molar has been partially by-passed). The teeth have been restored with well-fitting cast restorations. The treatment in both cases can be classified as a success as there has been complete regeneration of the periradicular tissues.

success rate may be as high as initial root treatment of the root canal space—as long as there is no evidence of chronic periradicular periodontitis.

Failure to eliminate microorganisms adequately, allowing their proliferation, or re-infection of the disinfected root canal space are the principal factors that may adversely affect the prognosis of root canal treatment.

Factors that have a secondary influence on outcome

It is difficult to compare the specific impact of the various aspects of canal preparation (e.g. instrumentation techniques, irrigation, and inter-appointment medicament regimes) and obturation on the prognosis of root canal

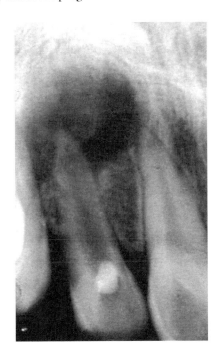
(a)

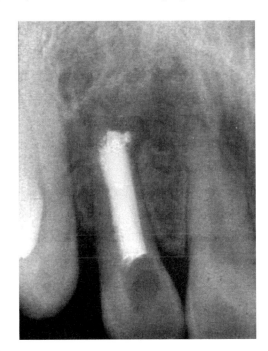
(b)

Fig. A7.9 (a) Very large periradicular lesion; (b) showing healing over time.

treatment from published studies, as there is poor standardization of methodology between these studies. This results in too many variables to allow the impact of individual factors on the prognosis of root canal treatment to be adequately assessed. What can be said is that the processes mentioned in Chapters A5 and A6 for disinfecting and sealing the root canal space appear to be effective in eliminating and preventing apical periodontitis.

Factors that have no influence on outcome

General factors

There is no conclusive evidence to suggest that age, sex or medical problems that the patient may be suffering from have an influence on the prognosis of treatment.

Size of pre-operative radiolucency

The size of the pre-operative lesion does not affect the prognosis of the treatment, but larger lesions will take a longer time period to heal completely and Figs A7.9(a) and (b)).

Conclusion

In summary, it is clear that successful root canal treatment revolves around *eliminating and preventing (re-)infection* of the root canal space. The role of microorganisms in the determination of a successful outcome cannot be overemphasized.

Dealing with failure

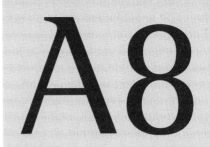

Dealing with failure

Understanding failure

All dental practitioners would like to be able to achieve successful treatment outcomes for their patients. Even though endodontic procedures have relatively high success rates compared with other dental disciplines, it is unwise to guarantee a perfect result even when procedures have been performed with the greatest of care. Patients should be warned in advance of the possible risks that accompany treatment, even though these may be slight. Failure is something that everyone faces at various times during a professional career. It is important to be able to understand the mechanisms of failure so that failure might be recognized and dealt with in an appropriate fashion. Further, learning should occur from instances of failure and systems be put in place to limit its recurrence.

It has been emphasized repeatedly that the presence of microorganisms is the primary causative factor in failure.

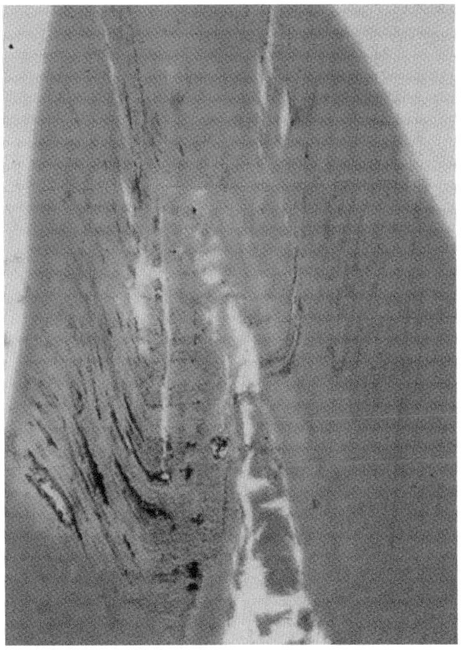

The presence of microorganisms in the root canal system may be explained in three ways:

- The microorganisms might have been left within the pulp space during the previous endodontic treatment (Fig. A8.1). These residual microbes, should they sur-

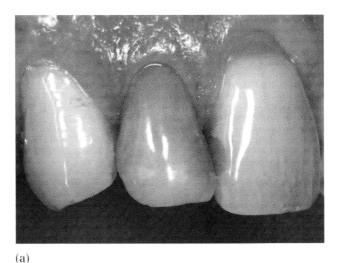

(a)

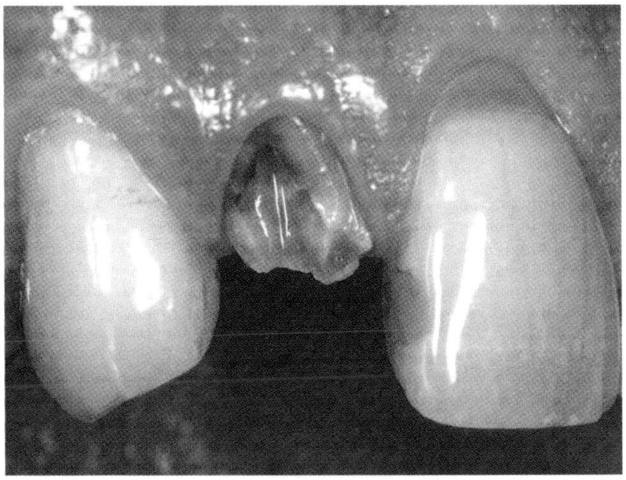

(b)

Fig. A8.2 (a) Root-treated lateral incisor; (b) lateral incisor following fracture—note discolouration of dentine due to coronal leakage.

Fig. A8.1 Residual microorganisms in dentinal tubules.

vive and proliferate, are likely to produce toxins that have an effect upon the immune system of the host and lead to pathological changes. These changes may become evident clinically or radiographically;

♦ The microorganisms may have re-entered the pulp space of the tooth following the obturation of the root canal system. The source of these contaminant organisms is the oral flora. The avenues for re-entry might include fractures and lack of sealing by coronal restorations (Fig. A8.2(a) and (b));

♦ Failure that occurs in teeth that have been apparently completely cleaned and obturated is always perplexing (Fig. A8.3). The continuing presence of the microorganisms, if not within unfilled lateral and accessory canals, may be explained by an ability of certain organisms to survive in the periradicular tissues or the periradicular cementum.

How is failure recognized?

The assessment of previous endodontic treatment should be based upon a sound history, signs, and symptoms reported by the patient and a thorough clinical and radiographic examination (Chapter A7). When failure is apparent, the cause needs to be clearly established before the future management of the situation can be decided upon.

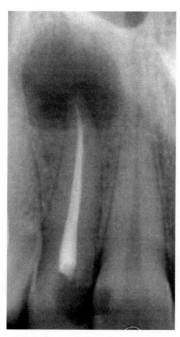

Fig. A8.3 Persistent lesion related to an apparently well-disinfected and obturated lateral incisor.

Relevant history

The history of previous treatment is valuable and every effort should be made to glean as much information as possible. In addition to the normal questions asked during the examination of all patients, the following questions might be considered:

♦ *Where was the treatment performed?* You may not have provided the treatment (for example, treatment may have been carried out in a hospital, general or specialist practice). It is always worth trying to establish the name and whereabouts of the operator.

♦ *What was the original diagnosis?* The patient may be in a position to provide information about the reason for the original treatment. It may be possible to distinguish between a pulpal or periradicular problem and whether or not there was radiographic evidence of a periradicular radiolucency.

♦ *Was there any discomfort before, during or immediately after treatment?* The patient may be in a position to remember both the timing and the nature of any pain experienced. The likelihood of complications during treatment may be identified.

♦ *What techniques were used during the treatment?* Patients remember the use of rubber dam and the taking of radiographs. They may not remember the names of irrigants and medicaments but they may be able to describe the odours associated with their use. It should be possible to obtain some idea of the number of appointments and the amount of time devoted to the treatment.

Examination

It is very important to look for all signs of endodontic disease. As already mentioned, the absence of symptoms is not necessarily an indicator of the absence of disease. The clinical appearance of swellings and sinuses may be indicative of failure and radiographs are of particular use.

Periapical radiographs should be checked for signs of periradicular pathology. Radiographs of root fillings do not tell a great deal about the biological state of the teeth. A 'nice'-looking root filling does not guarantee the absence of infection. The root canal(s) may in fact contain a multitude of microorganisms. An up-to-date periapical radiograph only gives a two-dimensional image of the current status of a tooth. Such radiographs fail to give accurate information about previous treatment and the events that have occurred since treatment. Where previous radiographs are available, they should also be examined to identify possible changes in the radiographic appearance of the supporting tissues. Where previous radiographs are not present and there are no symptoms, it may be wise to re-assess matters in another 6–12 months so that comparisons can be drawn.

What are the treatment options?

When failure has been diagnosed, the suspected cause should be determined. The cause of failure is related primarily to the presence of microorganisms. The choice of treatment is made on the basis of the strategic importance of the tooth, procedural complexities, operator ability, patient preferences, motivation and cost. The main treatment options to consider are:

- no treatment;
- extraction;
- re-root canal treatment;
- endodontic surgery.

No treatment

There are clinical situations where there are indications that the treatment has not been a total success but the situation is stable enough to consider review rather than interceptive treatment. This can often be the case in teeth that were treated many years ago and have remained symptomless. Close examination reveals that there exists a chronic periradicular periodontitis that is not completely healed but has remained dormant for some time (Fig. A8.4).

Active treatment may carry certain risks e.g. root fracture and complications that are best avoided until there are positive signs of deterioration. Such teeth may require monitoring and treatment should be considered at an appropriate time.

An example of such a scenario might be a symptomless, crowned tooth with a stable chronic lesion. Treatment of the lesion might be deferred until such time that the crown needs to be replaced. Where a decision is made to merely observe the progress of a treatment failure, the patient must be warned of the possibility of an unexpected flare-up.

Extraction

There are situations where extraction might be the most suitable treatment. It should be remembered that extraction still remains the most expedient method of treating endodontic disease! With the extraction of the tooth, the microorganisms are eradicated and no longer have an effect on the host defence mechanisms. Extraction might be considered for teeth that are no longer functional or recognized to have untreatable complications. Such complications include vertical fractures or recurrent caries resulting in irreparable and extensive damage to the structure of the tooth, resulting in the tooth being unrestorable (Fig. A8.5).

Re-root canal treatment

Where the reasons for failure centre on clinically demonstrable treatment inadequacies, the treatment of choice should be conservative (non-surgical) retreatment. If doubts exist about the quality of the previous endodontic treatment then the treatment should be redone (revised).

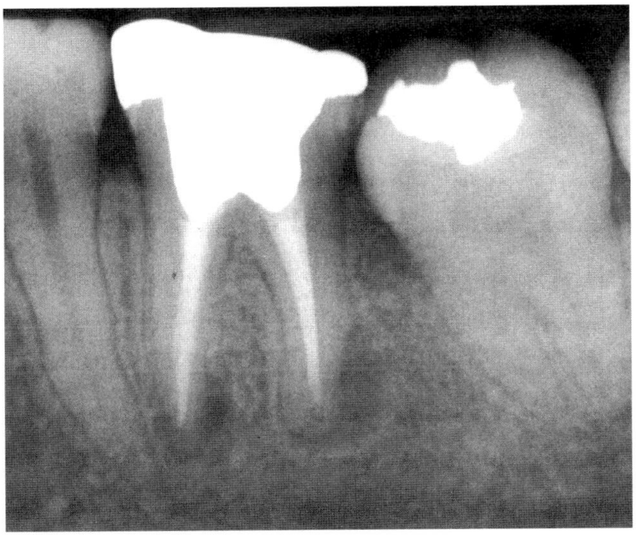

Fig. A8.4 Radiograph of a tooth that has remained symptomless with a periradicular radiolucency for many years.

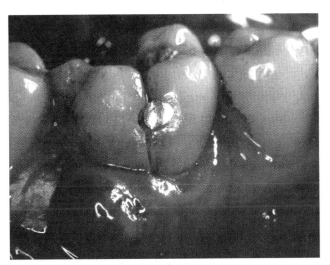

Fig. A8.5 An endodontically treated molar with a vertical root fracture that now requires extraction. If this tooth had been restored with a cast cuspal coverage restoration after root canal treatment, it might not have fractured.

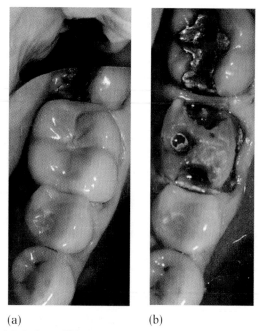

(a)   (b)

Fig. A8.6 (a and b) A crown is removed to assess if there is sufficient sound coronal tooth tissue for the provison of a new crown prior to the commencement of root canal treatment.

Endodontic retreatment is complicated by the presence of an obturating material in the pulp space. Fortunately, most endodontic materials can be removed from teeth using a combination of solvents and mechanical techniques. The presence of expensive coronal restorations can further complicate the retreatment. You are required to understand the methods available for the disassembly of these endodontically treated and restored teeth. The removal of coronal restorations, posts and obturating materials becomes an integral part of the retreatment procedures (see the accompanying Chapter B8).

Crown removal

Failure is commonly related to coronal leakage and recurrent caries. Old crowns may need to be removed and provisional restorations may be required to maintain the integrity of the tooth during treatment. A decision has to be made to either remove the crown or to cut an access cavity through it. This decision is made on the basis of the condition of the restoration and the overall treatment plan. The advantage of crown removal is that it allows an assessment of the condition of the underlying tooth substance and its restorability (Fig. A8.6(a) and (b)).

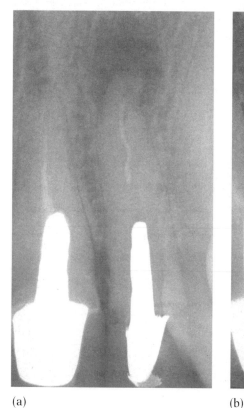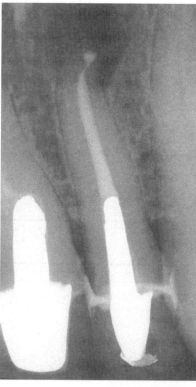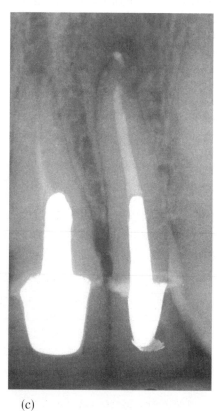

(a)   (b)   (c)

Fig. A8.7 (a) Lateral incisor restored with a cast post and core restoration—note the evidence of a periradicular lesion; (b) tooth re-treated following removal of the post crown (using ultrasonics); (c) radiographic evidence of resolving lesion 6 months later.

Post removal

The removal of posts can be a difficult and hazardous process. The risk of root fracture is an ever-present consideration that can be avoided by using the right equipment. Assessment should be made with the following factors in mind:

◆ the length and width of the post;

◆ the post design—parallel, tapered, or threaded;

◆ type of cement and possible history of previous de-cementation;

◆ aesthetic requirements particularly in relation to provisional restorations;

◆ patient wishes and cost.

Once the restoration and post have been successfully removed the tooth may be retreated in a conventional manner (Fig. A8.7(a)–(c)).

Removal of obturating materials

Gutta percha is the most commonly used material for the obturation of root canals. It is usually relatively easy to remove with the aid of solvents, the most commonly used of which are chloroform and eucalyptus oil. There are many techniques that may be adopted for the removal of GP. A combination of mechanical, thermal, and chemical activity seems to produce the desired result.

Silver points may be removed from root canals using ultrasonically activated tips or fine forceps. It is often necessary to remove dentine from around the coronal aspect of a silver point to allow the forceps room to grasp it. Examination of the example demonstrated confirms the removal of dentine (Fig. A8.8(a) and (b)).

Endodontic surgery

Surgical techniques have traditionally been used to deal with failing endodontic cases. Sadly, the surgical approach to these problems does not always deal with the coronal entry of microorganisms into the teeth. Endodontic surgery should therefore be considered as a 'last resort' when endeavouring to rectify obvious failure. The prognosis for teeth treated by surgery depends heavily on an ability to eradicate microorganisms and their products from the root canal systems of teeth. The positive indications for surgery are few and can be classified as follows:

◆ when it is impossible to gain access to the apical region of a tooth by conventional means—apical obstructions, well-fitting post crown restorations, calcified canals and insoluble endodontic materials may create this situation;

◆ when there is a need to perform a biopsy;

◆ where corrective measures require a surgical approach —this is particularly important in the treatment of perforations.

Surgery may also be contemplated where there is a persistent periradicular lesion despite high-quality conservative endodontic treatment that cannot be improved (Fig. A8.9). These types of cases should be referred for specialist treatment.

There are occasions when it is either impossible to remove a post-retained restoration or it is not convenient to do so. This may be the case following a recent extensive and expensive course of restorative treatment.

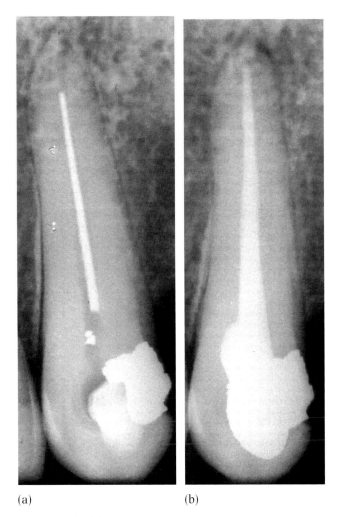

(a)   (b)

Fig. A8.8 (a) Silver point requiring removal from a canine; (b) canine retreated—note removal of coronal dentine to facilitate the removal of the silver point.

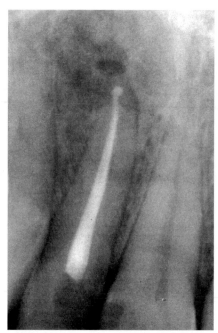

Fig. A8.9 Healing of the case demonstrated in Fig. A8.3 following endodontic surgery.

What are the main objectives of surgical treatment?

The main objectives of surgery remain similar to non-surgical procedures, namely the disinfection and sealing of the apical root canal system. Various materials have been employed to achieve effective seals. Materials used should be compatible with the oral tissues, readily adaptable to the root, and non-resorbable.

Various materials have been used over the years. These include dental amalgam, zinc oxide-based materials, glass ionomer, resins, and Mineral Trioxide Aggregate. Preference has moved away from amalgam towards zinc oxide-based materials (super EBA® and IRM®) and subsequently, Mineral Trioxide Aggregate (MTA®) has been used to achieve the required seal.

Referring patients

One of the most difficult situations to deal with is the failure to appreciate when one's own clinical experience and ability is insufficient to deal with the needs and demands of a patient. When expectations are beyond one's ability, referral must always be considered. Referral may be based not just on technical considerations but may be related to general patient management and costs. Ideally, it is better to identify potential difficulties before commencing treatment so that the patient can be referred to a more experienced colleague, who can then start and complete the procedure. Patients often prefer to have matters dealt with by one person. There are occasions when referral may be required during treatment when clinical situations become unmanageable. These include irresolvable pain, acute exacerbations, procedural accidents (for example, separated instruments and canal aberrations) or the inability to locate root canals.

Clear communication with the patient and the individual to whom the referral has been made should be conducted in a manner that prevents any misunderstanding. A written description of the predicament and treatment performed along with accompanying radiographs should be forwarded to the specialist in the form of a referral letter that explains the problem and the background to the referral.

This chapter concludes Section A on the theory and science of endodontology. Section B will provide a very practical guide to the clinical techniques of endodontics. It begins with 'Diagnosis, treatment planning, and patient management'. You are advised to refer back to this section whenever you feel it relevant to do so. The colour-coding system has been designed to try to help you achieve this.

Section B

Clinical, practical aspects

Diagnosis, treatment planning and patient management

Diagnosis, treatment planning and patient management

Introduction

Diagnosis and treatment planning are dependent upon relevant information being gained from the history elicited from a patient, the detailed examination and the selection, use and interpretation of special tests. Patient management is essential to the success of any planned treatment. The second part of this chapter covers some of the rudiments of successful treatment planning.

How do we take a history?

It is essential that the clinician is attentive, sympathetic and interested in the patient's presenting complaints. This will result in the patient being more inclined to provide a full account of their experiences. It is useful to have a mental checklist of the type of questions to ask that cover the nature and character of the presenting complaint. Some questions that might form the criteria for successful endodontic history taking are:

- 'What's the trouble? How may I help?'
- 'When did you first notice the problem?'
- 'How long have you had pain?'
- 'What does the pain feel like (sharp, dull, throbbing etc.)?'
- 'What starts the pain?'
- 'Where is the pain?'
- 'How long does the pain last?'
- 'When does it hurt most?'
- 'What makes the pain better?'.

It is advisable to always ask questions that do not require the answers 'yes' or 'no'. By doing this, it is possible to avoid putting words and descriptions into the patient's mind.

Dental history

Criteria for successful dental history taking are:

- 'When was the last time you saw the dentist?'
- 'How regularly do you attend?
- 'How many times a day do you brush/clean between your teeth?'
- 'How many spoonfuls of sugar do you have in your tea/coffee and how many cups do you drink a day?'
- 'Do you have a "sweet tooth"?'
- 'Have you ever knocked your front teeth?'
- 'Have you had recent dental treatment' (if so what/where/when/from whom?).

Medical history

Use a medical history questionnaire (*consult standard texts for this*). It is essential to gain information about medical conditions or potential complications that may influence endodontic treatment, for example, the need for antibiotic prophylaxis before treatment (see Fig. B3.1) or patients with adreno-cortical suppression due to steroid medication who may require steroid cover.

Extra-oral examination

The criteria for successful extraoral examination include assessment for:

- asymmetry (Fig. B3.2a);
- swelling/lymphadenopathy (see Fig. A6.3);
- tenderness of muscles of mastication;
- tenderness of swellings/lymphadenitis;
- extra-oral sinus (Fig. B3.2b);
- temporo-mandibular joint tenderness/clicking/crepitus.

Detailed observations (for example, size, location, severity of any extraoral tenderness or swelling) and subsequent note taking are essential.

Under local anaesthetic

Where there is no allergy to penicillin and the patient has received no more than one dose of penicillin in the last month:

- amoxycillin 3 g orally, 1 hour before treatment.

If there is a penicillin allergy or the patient has had more than one dose of penicillin in the last month:

- clindamycin 600 mg orally, 1 hour before treatment.

Under general anaesthetic

Where there is no allergy to penicillin and the patient has received no more than one dose of penicillin in the last month and is not classified as at high risk:

- amoxycillin 1 g intravenously on induction, then amoxycillin 500 mg orally 6 hours later;

or

- amoxycillin 3 g orally 4 hours before induction, then amoxycillin 3 g orally as soon as possible after recovery.

If the patient is at high risk of infective endocarditis (for example, there is a history of a previous episode of endocarditis or they have prosthetic heart valves):

- amoxycillin 1 g intravenously + gentamycin 120 mg intravenously on induction, then amoxycillin 500 mg orally 6 hours later.

If there is a penicillin allergy or the patient has had more than one course of penicillin in the last month:

- vancomycin 1 g intravenously over 100 min, then gentamycin 120 mg intravenously on induction (or 15 min pre-operatively).

NB: These are all adult dosages.

1. Stress the importance of maintenance of good oral hygiene.

2. Use chlorhexidine mouthwash to reduce oral bacterial level prior to treatment.

3. Make a value judgement about the role and effectiveness of root canal treatment in all cases, particularly where antibiotic cover is indicated in the high-risk category of the medically compromised patient.

Fig. B3.1 Suggested antibiotic prophylaxis for patients at risk of infective endocarditis. Always refer to the BNF.

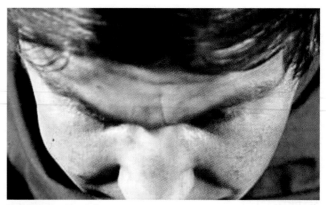

Fig. B3.2a Facial asymmetry.

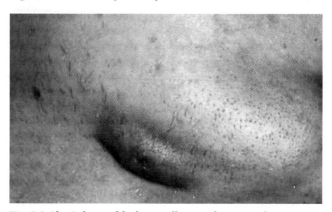

Fig. B3.2b Submandibular swelling and extraoral sinus.

Intra-oral examination

The criteria for successful intra-oral examination can be broken down into the following stages:

Access

- Assess interincisor distance—is there adequate access for you to comfortably assess the tooth and if necessary, treat it (Fig. A3.5)?

- Can the patient open their mouth wide reasonably comfortably for a long period of time?

- Is the patient comfortable in the supine position?

- Does the patient have a pronounced gag reflex, i.e. can they tolerate the positioning of intra-oral posterior X-ray film holders?

General examination

General examination should check for the following:

- abnormal appearance of the oral mucosa (sinus, ulceration and erythema);

- frictional keratosis/scalloping of tongue;

- presence, location, tenderness, consistency and size of soft tissue abnormalities and swellings;

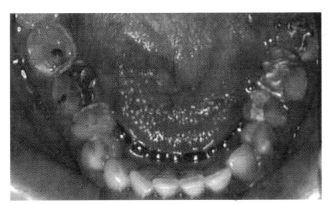

Fig. B3.3 Marked tooth surface loss may affect the integrity of the pulp.

- basic periodontal examination;
- plaque-retentive factors (Fig. A3.9(a) and (b));
- tooth surface loss (Fig. B3.3);
- food trapping (Fig. B3.4a);
- quality of existing dental treatment/restorations.
- caries/signs of marginal leakage (Figs. A2.16 and A3.14);
- fractured teeth and restorations (Fig. B3.4b);
- discolouration of teeth (Figs. A2.28 and A3.3(a)).

Detailed examination of the area of main complaint

A detailed examination of the area(s) of discomfort should be carried out. Examination of the colour and consistency of any swelling (see Fig. A3.10) (rubbery/firm/fluctuant) of the related soft and hard tissues will help in formulating a diagnosis. A note should be made of any abnormal appearance of the mucosa overlying the area in question (for example, presence of a sinus tract or erythema). A record of the size, location and texture of any swelling should be noted. The origin of any sinus tract should be traced with a gutta percha point and radiographed (see later). Diagrams or even photographs of the area in question may supplement note taking.

The next stage is to assess the alveolar region housing the tooth or teeth in question, after which the teeth are examined. The assessment should check for, or include:

- tenderness to palpation;
- tenderness to percussion;
- mobility;
- periodontal profile;
- fractured cusps;
- occlusal examination;
- assessment of teeth;
- discolouration of teeth.

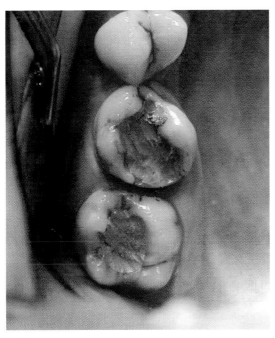

(a)

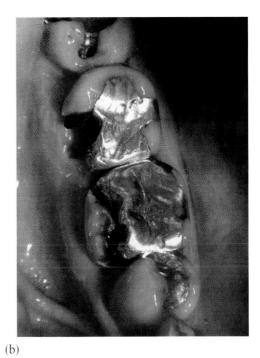

(b)

Fig. B3.4 (a) Open contact between teeth (in this case upper first and second molar teeth) may result in food packing interproximally, the symptoms of which may mimic pulpal disease; (b) fractured restorations.

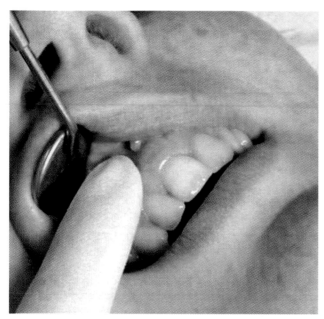

Fig. B3.5 Tenderness to palpation assessed by gently pressing the mucosa.

Palpation: The mucosa on either side of the area of complaint should be palpated gently using finger pressure only (Fig. B3.5). A note should be made of any tenderness to palpation along with the extent/severity of tenderness; the contralateral/adjacent quadrant should also be palpated to provide a comparison.

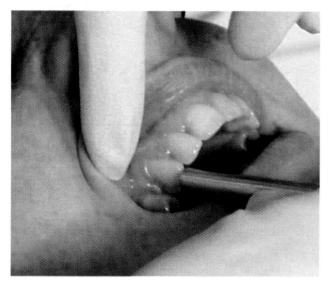

Fig. B3.6 Gentle percussion of a tooth with a mirror handle.

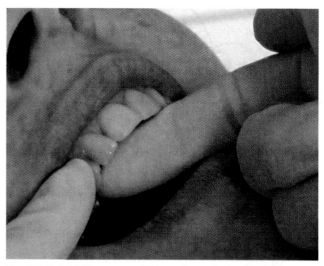

Fig. B3.7 Mobility assessed by applying fingertip pressure to the labial and palatal aspects of the crown of the tooth.

Percussion: Gently tapping the tooth with a fingertip may result in a transient or sometimes a prolonged tenderness, but it may be easier to elicit any tenderness to percussion by gently tapping on the tooth with the end of a mirror handle (Fig. B3.6). It is important to tap each cusp tip (and therefore each root) if a posterior tooth is being assessed, as only one root may be tender to percussion.

Mobility: Mobility of teeth should be noted and graded according to severity. The tooth should be placed between the fingertips and gently pressed buccally and then palatally (Fig. B3.7). A note should then be made of the mobility of the tooth (for example, grade I = less than 1 mm horizontal mobility, grade II = 1–2 mm horizontal movement, and grade III = vertical movement or more than 2 mm horizontal movement). It may be easier to use the end of mirror handles to assess the severity of mobility in some cases.

Periodontal probing: When probing the tooth, the periodontal probe should be 'walked' around the complete circumference of the tooth under investigation, as it is not uncommon to miss vertically fractured teeth (Fig. A3.11(a) and (b)).

Occlusal examination: This part of the clinical examination comprises:

◆ Assessing for signs of excess occlusal loading or trauma, parafunction and musculo-skeletal pain on the mucosa and teeth. Articulating paper may be used to identify points of premature contact (Fig. B3.8).

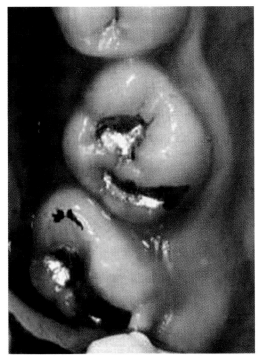

Fig. B3.8 Mark left on maxillary molar following the use of articulating paper to detect irregular points (e.g. non-working side interferences, high spots) of contact.

* Assessing teeth in retruded contact and intercuspal positions and then lateral excursions.

* Fracture detection: Incomplete coronal fractures play an important role in the spread of pulpal and periradicular disease. Their detection is achieved either by direct vision or the use of a 'wedge test' (Fig. B3.9(a) and (b)). The criteria for a successful examination are:

* good light and magnification; look for crazes, infractions, and hairline cracks;

* placing 'tooth slooth'/cut piece of rubber dam in artery clip holders over selected cusp;

* asking patient to close firmly;

* confirming which cusps tips are contacting;

* asking patient to open;

* noting if the patient's symptoms are reproduced when he/she closes, or opens from closed position.

Assessment of Teeth: During examination, an attempt should be made to imagine the amount of sound coronal

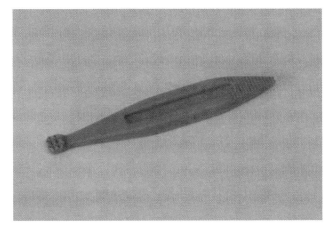

(a)

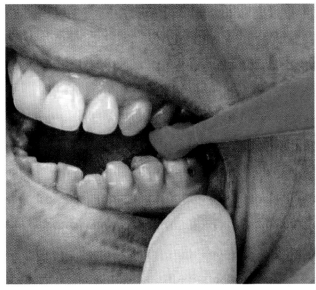

(b)

Fig. B3.9 (a) The 'tooth slooth'; (b) a 'tooth slooth' being used to reproduce symptoms of cracked tooth syndrome, which may be hard to localize for both the patient and the operator.

tooth that would remain after removal of caries and previous restorations. This should give a guide to the restorability of the tooth. Figure B3.10(a) and (b) shows a maxillary premolar before and after root canal treatment and coronal restoration. Endodontic treatment is futile when carried out for teeth that are unrestorable. When teeth appear restorable, the amount and position of remaining tooth tissue will influence the type of procedure performed for the construction of a post-treatment restoration.

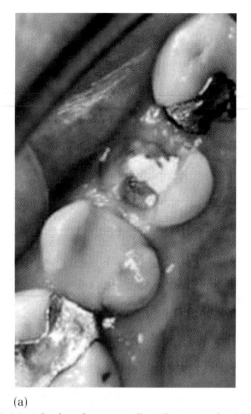

(a)

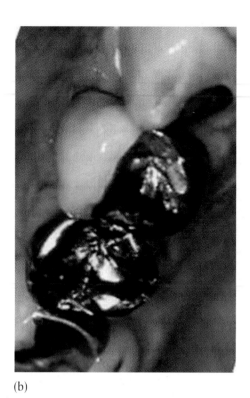

(b)

Fig. B3.10 A broken down maxillary first premolar (a) before and (b) after root canal treatment and restoration.

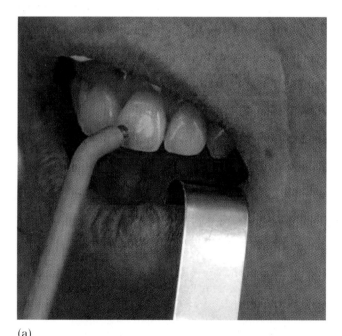

(a)

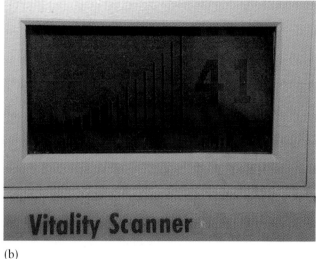

(b)

Fig. B3.11 (a) An electric pulp tester (Analytic Vitality Tester) in use, note the lip clip in the corner of the mouth to complete an electric circuit. (b) The digital display of the apex locator indicates the current applied to the tooth and the rate at which it has been set to increase.

Discoloured teeth: The following should be checked for:

* shade of discolouration;
* uniformity;
* extent(partially/totally discoloured).

Special investigations
Vitality testing

The following criteria are essential for predictable vitality testing (any method):

* advise patient of test and to raise their hand when they feel the stimulus;
* dry tooth to be tested with gauze and isolate with cotton pledgets;
* first test a healthy tooth;
* test tooth in question and record finding;
* attempt to test both the buccal and lingual/palatal aspects of multi-rooted teeth;
* repeat testing if necessary;
* test adjacent and contralateral teeth to gain more objective comparisons.

Electric pulp testing

The aim of this test is to make a local electrical circuit between the patient's oral mucosa and the tooth to be investigated. A small clip is hooked around the patient's lip and the probe is placed on the coronal half of the tooth in question to complete the circuit (Fig. B3.11). Alternatively, the patient completes the circuit by holding the handle of the electrode that contacts the tooth. A conducting medium such as toothpaste or prophylaxis paste between the tooth and probe is essential. The patient is asked to make a sign (for example, lifting of a hand) when they feel warmth or tingling on the tooth being investigated. The electric current passing through the tooth increases the longer the probe is left on the tooth. The rate at which the current increases may be adjusted.

Cold testing

A cold stimulus such as dichloro-difluoro-methane refrigerant spray, e.g. Endo-Frost® (approximately −5°C) is sprayed onto a cotton pledget and applied to the tooth under investigation. Ethyl chloride (−4°C) (Fig. B3.12a) is a common alternative but it may be considered insufficiently discriminatory (giving rise to false negatives) as it is not as cold as Endo-Frost®. Ice sticks may also be used for the same purpose.

Heat testing

Teeth may be isolated, individually, with rubber dam and hot water applied via a syringe to the tooth under investigation (Fig. A3.19(b)). Alternatively a GP stick may be heated and then applied to the tooth but a separating medium such as Vaseline should be coated sparingly on to the tooth to ensure that the GP does not stick to the enamel (Fig. B3.12b).

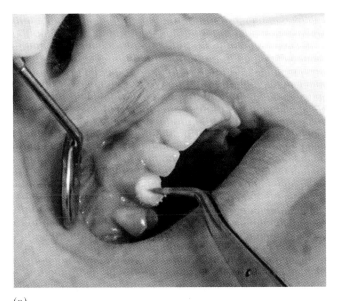

(a)

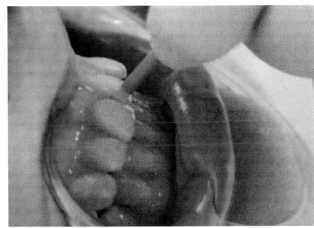

(b)

Fig. B3.12 (a) Ethyl chloride being applied to a tooth using a cotton pledget. **(b)** heated gutta percha stick applied to tooth.

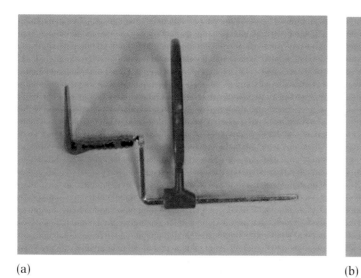

(a)

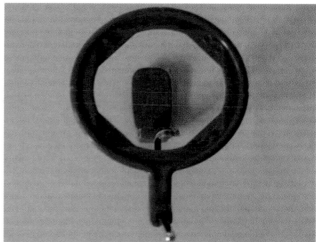

(b)

Fig. B3.13 Anterior Rinn® film holder: (a) side view; (b) end on.

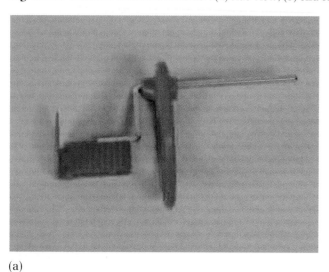

(a)

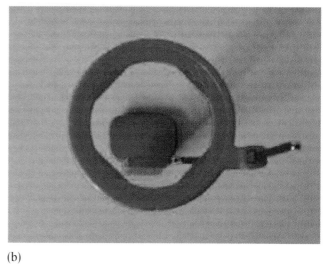

(b)

Fig. B3.14 Posterior film holder: (a) side view; (b) end on.

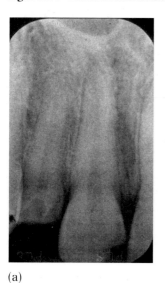

(a)

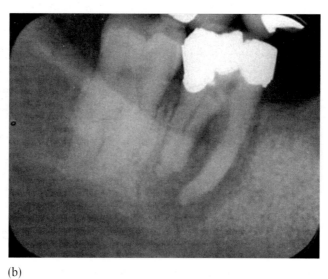

(b)

Fig. B3.15 Radiographs taken using a paralleling device: (a) anterior; (b) posterior.

Test cavity preparation

In extreme cases, a cavity is prepared in a tooth under copious irrigation with no local anaesthetic, using a sharp bur. The patient should be advised to make a signal if or when they feel any sensation. If the tooth is necrotic the bur will eventually access the pulp chamber with no discomfort.

Radiographic examination

All aspects of endodontic practice are heavily reliant upon information gained from radiographs. Radiographs are taken pre-operatively, during treatment and post-operatively.

Periapical radiographs

The criteria for success are as follows:

- X-ray film should be in a paralleling device. These devices are designed for use in anterior [(Fig. B3.13(a) and (b)] and posterior [(Fig. B3.14(a) and (b)] teeth;

- The radiograph should show the complete tooth together with at least 3–4 mm of surrounding bone (Fig. B3.15(a) and (b));

- The following features should be assessed:

  - the radiodensity of the associated alveolar bone;

  - the integrity of the 'lamina dura';

  - the continuity of the periodontal ligament space and any widening of it;

  - the presence of a periradicular radiolucency;

  - the length of the root;

  - the number of roots and their degree of curvature;

- the root canal anatomy of the tooth including pulp space contents, for example, pulp stones and tertiary dentine;

- any abrupt loss of root canal outline (which may indicate the bifurcation of one canal into two root canals);

- the presence, type and quality of previous root canal treatment;

- coronal and root caries;

- state of the coronal restoration.

If there is an intra- or extraoral sinus, valuable information can be secured by placing a GP point in the sinus tract. A periapical radiograph is then taken to reveal the origins of the infection (Fig. B3.16(a) and (b)).

Parallax views

The use of two periapical views taken at slightly different horizontal angles has already been mentioned (Fig. A3.21(a) and (b)). A horizontal shift of the tube angle of about 10° to take a second radiograph (Fig. B3.17(a) and (b)) may produce a more revealing image of the tooth under investigation (Fig. B3.18(a) and (b)).

Arriving at a diagnosis

Whist it is a straightforward process to read books that list the processes required to achieve accurate diagnoses, the reality is complex. It requires experience and practise to assimilate the many (often conflicting) pieces of information whilst sieving and prioritizing information. Remember that the skill of critical reasoning or of processing information takes time

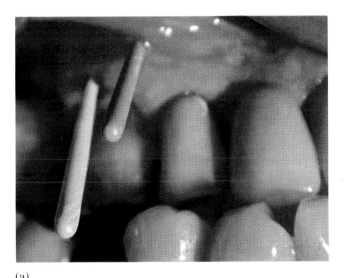

(a)

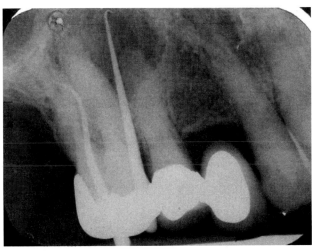

(b)

Fig. B3.16 Two gutta percha points have been used to 'track' patent sinuses: (a) clinical view; (b) periapical radiograph.

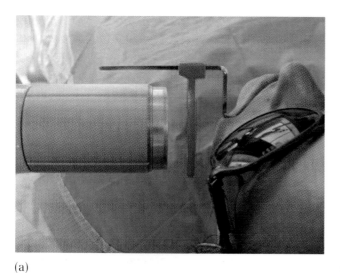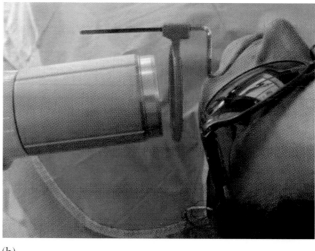

(a) (b)

Fig. B3.17 Two periapical views are taken: (a) straight on; (b) with a horizontal shift of 10° to the distal.

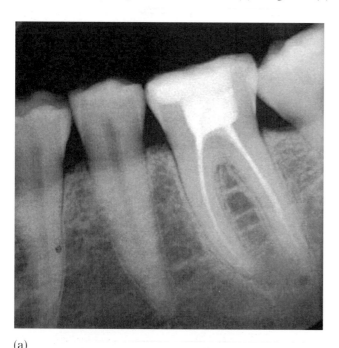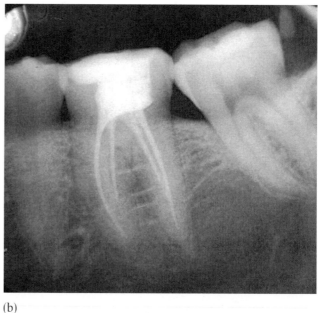

(a) (b)

Fig. B3.18 Parallax radiographs of the mandibular molar (a) straight on and (b) with a horizontal shift of 10° reveal additional canals.

to learn. Below is a brief summary of the common points that you need to rationalize in endodontic diagnosis:

- reason for attendance
- presenting complaint and its history
- dental, family and social history
- medical history
- extraoral examination
- intraoral examination
  - mucosa
  - supporting tissues of teeth (basic periodontal examination)
  - general appraisal of dentition
  - detailed assessment of tooth or teeth in question
  - occlusion and occlusal relationships
- special tests and investigations
  - vitality tests
  - radiographs (for example, paralleling periapical films of teeth under investigation).

Diagnosis

Crucial to endodontic diagnosis is the relationship between symptoms, signs and histopathological pulpal state. Unfortunately, these relationships are not clearly defined or reproducible but you should read Chapter A2 again for pointers that will aid investigation. Before proceeding, you should confirm that you are able to provide a summary statement (presenting symptoms, clinical and radiographic signs and treatment options for each of the diagnoses below:

- reversible pulpitis;
- irreversible pulpitis;
- acute periradicular periodontitis;
- acute periradicular abscess;
- chronic periradicular periodontitis;
- chronic periradicular periodontitis with an associated sinus.

What are the common errors in diagnosis?

Endodontic disease usually manifests itself clinically in the form of pain, swelling and/or periapical radiolucency. However, the clinician should always be aware that there are non-endodontic aetiologies for pain, swelling and periradicular radiolucency (detailed explanations are provided in standard texts on oral medicine and oral pathology).

Radiographic errors

In symptomless situations, the only sign of endodontic disease may be periradicular radiolucency and the operator may only notice such a finding on a routine radiograph (for example, an infected necrotic root canal associated with chronic periradicular periodontitis) (Fig. B3.19a). However, it should be remembered that certain 'silent' radiographic lesions may be anatomically in close association with teeth but may not be of odontogenic origin (e.g. anatomical landmarks like the mental foramen) (Fig. B3.19b).

Alternatively, radiographic examination may reveal a radiographic lesion not related to the patient's perceived problems but in the region of the reported problem area; this may be attributed wrongly to the symptoms or clinical findings. This will result in a misdiagnosis being made and possibly inappropriate treatment.

You should be able to arrive at a differential diagnosis for radiographic lesions detected (more commonly radiolucent than radiopaque) depending on their location, size, shape, radiodensity, outline and effect on neighbouring structures (Fig. B3.20). Examples of errors that occur when over-reliance is placed on radiographic findings include the following:

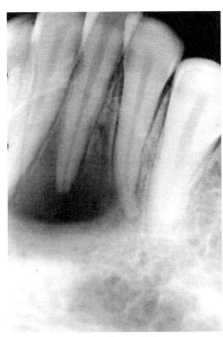

Fig. B3.19a Large periradicular radiolucency associated with symptomless teeth.

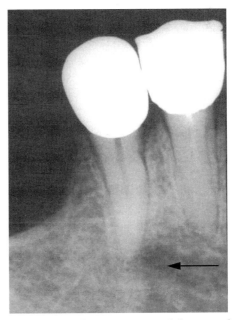

Fig. B3.19b Radiographic appearance of the mental foramen can be confusing when the endodontic health of teeth is suspect.

Radiolucent lesions

- normal anatomy (mental foramen)
- artefactual (processing errors)
- pathological
  - infection
  - trauma
  - cyst
  - tumour/tumour-like lesion
  - giant cell lesion
  - fibro-cemento-osseous lesion.

Swellings

- abscess of odontogenic origin
- cysts (odontogenic commoner than non-odontogenic)
- odontogenic tumours
- giant cell lesions
- fibro-osseous lesions
- non-odontogenic neoplasms of bone.

Fig. B3.20 Differential diagnosis of radiolucent lesions/swelling.

Anatomical landmarks

Mental and incisive foramina may be mistaken for radiolucent lesions associated with infected necrotic pulps. Vitality testing will help confirm that these 'radiolucencies' are anatomical landmarks. Radiographs (e.g. panoramic views) show the contralateral side and would also confirm the position of the mental foramen to be in a similar location. Widening of the periodontal ligament space and apparent radiolucencies may be due to superimposition of root apices over the maxillary sinuses and inferior dental canal. Sparse bony trabeculation may also be mistaken for a pathological lesion.

Periapical cemental-osseous dysplasia

These lesions are usually associated with the apices of mandibular incisor teeth and may be mistaken for periradicular lesions. Vitality testing and even follow-up radiographs will confirm that the area is harmless.

Non-inflammatory swellings

Although non-inflammatory swellings have unique presenting features, in reality the range of their presenting features does not preclude their occasional and passing resemblance to those of periradicular origin. You should be familiar with these conditions and their characteristics and be on guard to differentiate among them. The details of such diseases are covered comprehensively in more appropriate texts. A summary is provided in Fig. B3.20.

Once a differential diagnosis has been achieved, treatment planning may ensue. As described in Chapter A3, successful treatment planning is based on the appropriate choice of treatment strategies dependent upon the individual patient's needs and wishes. Section C of this book provides some clinical scenarios that mimic treatment-planning decision making.

Patient management

A brief resumé of issues that may be pertinent to patient management in the course of endodontic treatment is provided to stimulate thought and reflection for action. It is not comprehensive but is based on common situations that may present to you whilst inexperienced. The criteria presented are not often found in texts on endodontics and are presented to stimulate discussion.

Local anaesthesia

Good anaesthetic technique is an essential stage of root canal treatment, as without it patient confidence and trust may be lost. A significant number of patients are very nervous of having dental treatment due to painful treatment in the past, resulting from inadequate anaesthesia. This is a relatively common reason for some patients to delay seeing the dentist.

The criteria for successful local anaesthesia are as follows:

- decide on local anaesthetic technique and type of local anaesthetic to be used;
- apply topical anaesthetic to area to be injected;
- warm anaesthetic cartridges to body temperature;
- give injections slowly using a self-aspirating syringe;
- confirm adequate anaesthesia has been achieved *before* starting treatment by gently probing the mucosa in the area that has been anaesthetized;
- advise patient to raise a hand if they feel any pain (advise them that it is normal to feel pressure and vibration);
- start treatment.

Many factors affect administration and the effect of local anaesthesia. You need to be aware of the mechanism of action of various local anaesthetics, methods of adminis-

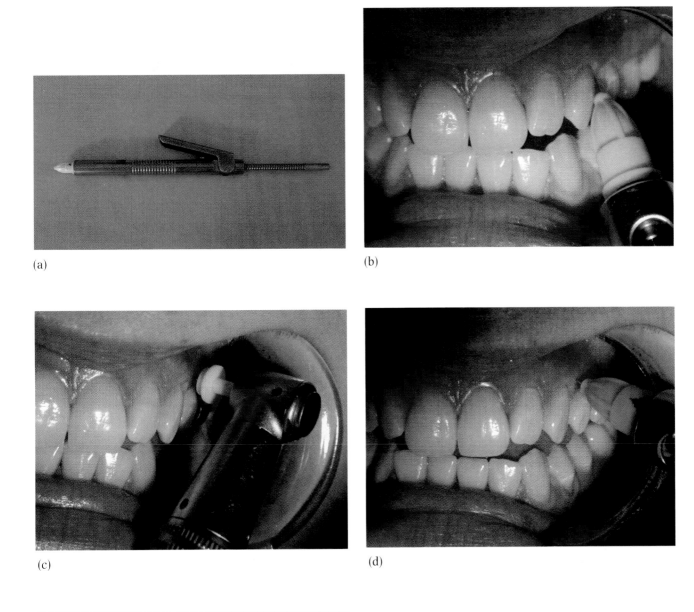

(a)

(b)

(c)

(d)

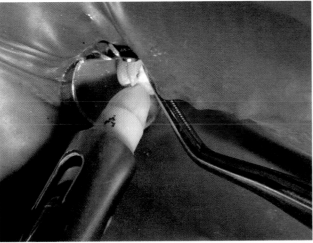

(e)

Fig. B3.21 (a) Parojet® for intraligamental injection; (b) needle placed along the long axis of the root for intraligamental injection; (c) intraosseous (Stabident®) system, a slow speed contra-angle slow handpiece with a perforator penetrating cortical plate; (d) needle (identical gauge to perforator) introduced into drill hole created by perforator; (e) intrapulpal injection-needle inserted into inflamed pulp tissue with cotton pledget sealing the remaining access cavity thus allowing local anaesthetic solution to be injected into pulp under pressure.

tration, and factors that modulate effectiveness. For maxillary teeth, an infiltration technique into the buccal mucosa adjacent to the roots of the tooth to be treated may be adequate. However, it is advisable to consider supplementing the customary buccal infiltration with a palatal infiltration.

Infiltration techniques to anaesthetize premolar and molar teeth are rarely successful in the mandible due to the thickness of the cortical bone. It is advisable to use an inferior dental block, which may be supplemented with the mental block for lower anterior teeth. The inferior dental block may also be supplemented with injections to anaesthetize the long buccal nerve.

If these techniques are not successful, additional anaesthetic techniques (Fig. B3.21) may be required, but always seek guidance from a *clinical tutor* before proceeding with further injections:

- regional nerve blocks (for maxillary teeth);
- intraligamental (Fig. B3.21a–b);
- Intraosseous (Fig. B3.21c–d);
- Intrapulpal (Fig. B3.21e).

Texts on local anaesthesia will provide the necessary information.

In extreme circumstances, despite competent use of a variety of local anaesthetic techniques, it may still not be possible to achieve adequate anaesthesia (see Box B3.1). In these cases, intravenous sedation may be considered. Light oral sedation (for example, 10 mg of diazepam) or nitrous oxide may be advisable for overly anxious patients prior to commencing treatment.

Patients may still be in some discomfort after (emergency) treatment has been completed, especially if they have presented reporting that they were taking analgesics for pain relief prior to root canal treatment.

Patients should always be advised that it is normal to be in some discomfort for several days after root canal treatment and therefore they should be given pain relief advice (see later). A telephone call from the dentist to enquire how the patient is 1–2 days after treatment is recommended, as it will be of tremendous psychological benefit to the patient.

A non-steroidal anti-inflammatory drug (NSAID) such as Ibuprofen is the first drug of choice. If this is not completely effective it may be supplemented with paracetamol or codeine phosphate/paracetamol preparations (e.g. Solpadeine®). These should be introduced 4 hours after the NSAID, therefore maximizing their efficacy. However, these analgesics should only be taken once it has been confirmed that the medication will not interfere with the patient's medical history. Very rarely, a stronger opioid may have to be prescribed if the pain relief from the over-the-counter analgesics is ineffective.

Vital pulp extirpation

Extirpation is indicated when the pulp is irreversibly inflamed. Profound anaesthesia is required for successful extirpation and unfortunately, it is sometimes difficult to achieve this to a satisfactory degree due to the extent of inflammation. Supplemental anaesthetic techniques may be required (as mentioned above) and it is essential to advise the patient that they may feel discomfort or pain during the procedure.

In addition, such cases tend to present as emergency appointments, when the dentist has little allocated time and is under pressure to provide effective treatment quickly.

The criteria for the success of vital extirpation are:

- paralleling periapical radiograph;
- profound local analgesia;
- rubber dam;
- access tooth and locate canal system;
- copious irrigation;
- as much preparation as possible in the time available;
- copious irrigation;
- Ledermix® intracanal dressing, if necessary;
- cotton wool and temporary seal;
- analgesic advice;
- appointment for definitive treatment.

Incisional drainage

A localized swelling, if not adequately treated, may progress through the cortical plate and spread along the soft tissue fascial planes (Fig. A6.3), through bone

---

- poor operator technique
- inadequate amounts of local anaesthetic administered
- variation in patient's anatomy
- very inflamed tissue/bone being anesthetized
- variation in absorption, metabolism and excretion of local anaesthetic solution
- psychological factors.

Box B3.1 Reasons for failure of anaesthesia.

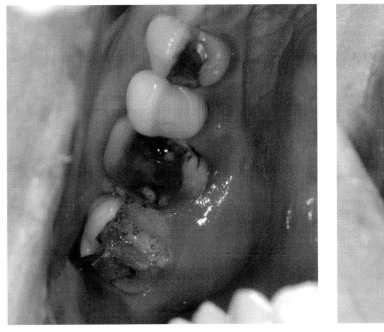 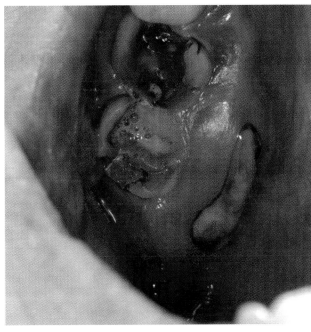

(a)   (b)

Fig. B3.22 (a) Palatal fluctuant swelling associated with an infected necrotic molar tooth; (b) the swelling has been lanced allowing drainage of pus.

(osteomyelitis), or via the bloodstream (bacteraemia). Patients presenting with an intraoral or extraoral swelling must be treated as a matter of urgency. In extreme cases the swelling may result in life-threatening conditions (Ludwig's angina, septicaemia). An attempt must be made to drain the contents of the swelling (abscess). This may be readily achievable through the soft tissues in cases where the swelling is fluctuant (Fig. B3.22). In addition, drainage via the root canals (see Fig. A2.29) should also be attempted. Adequate drainage will result in immediate pain relief and a reduction in the size of the swelling. Administration of local anaesthetic directly into the affected area is contraindicated in these situations as first, it may spread the infection along the fascial planes and second, due to the acute localized inflammatory reaction in the tissue, the anaesthetic solution will not be very effective.

The criteria for successful drainage via root canal(s) are:

- support tooth to prevent vibration;

- access tooth and gain entry into root canal(s)—pus should drain;

- use copious irrigation;

- gently massage swelling with finger to express as much pus as possible though canal(s);

- once the abscess stops draining dress the tooth with calcium hydroxide and a temporary coronal seal;

- adjust the tooth out of occlusion;

- prescribe antibiotics if there are signs of systemic involvement;

- give supportive care advice (analgesics, plenty of fluids, and soft diet).

The criteria for successful drainage via intra-oral swelling are:

- palpate swelling to confirm that it is fluctuant (indicating that pus is present);

- apply topical anaesthetic or spray ethyl chloride over the most fluctuant part of swelling (usually has creamy white head);

- lance this area with the tip of scalpel blade;

- gently massage either side of swelling with fingers to express as much pus as possible though incision;

- prescribe antibiotics;

- give supportive care advice (analgesics, plenty of fluids, and soft diet).

Antibiotics (Box B3.2) must be prescribed if a patient presents with a diffuse swelling that cannot be adequately drained via the root canal(s) or by incision and drainage of the swelling. A raised temperature (usually in association with malaise) is another indication when antibiotics should be prescribed. It should be borne in mind that antibiotics limit the spread of the infection and do not adequately treat the abscess or aetiological cause of the problem. If the cause of the endodontic problem is identified and treated successfully (pulp extirpation), antibiotics may not be required.

If antibiotics are prescribed as the first line of treatment, this may result in temporary pain relief but you must be aware that the cause of the problem is still present. *You should also remember that the overzealous use of antibiotics for a 'quick fix' of symptoms is never the treatment option of choice and it may result in increased resistance of antibiotics (and decreased effectiveness).*

The criteria for the successful prescription of a course of antibiotics are:

- no other treatment can alleviate patient's symptoms and signs;

- signs of systemic infection present (increased temperature, swelling present);

- medical history checked to confirm that antibiotic would not interfere with other medication or complicate existing medical history (for example, allergies [penicillin], drug interaction [such as warfarin] and pregnancy);

- choose the antibiotic most suitable for the infection;

- prescribe adequate dose, duration and route of administration (usually orally);

- advise patient of any possible interactions or side-effects.

Preparatory treatment of broken-down tooth prior to endodontic treatment

It is not uncommon once posterior (premolar and molar) teeth have been dismantled (removal of existing restoration and associated caries) to discover inadequate coronal tooth structure on one (or more) aspect(s) of the tooth. This may result in it being impossible to obtain adequate isolation with rubber dam or to allow retention of an inter-appointment temporary coronal seal. In these cases it is strongly advisable to build up a provisional core prior to starting root canal treatment. The core may be built up with the aid of a matrix band, a suitably trimmed copper band or by the use of an orthodontic band cemented around the tooth (Fig. B3.23).

The criteria for successful pre-endodontic core restoration build-up with an orthodontic band are:

- remove all restorations and caries from tooth;

- select a well-fitting orthodontic band;

- place cotton pledget directly over canal orifices to prevent cement entering; make sure cotton pledget is well away from tooth margins;

- burnish gingival margins of the band;

- cement orthodontic band with luting cement;

- restore tooth with glass-ionomer cement;

- prepare access cavity, remove cotton pledget, and commence endodontic treatment.

Metronidazole (effective against anaerobic endodontic bacteria)

    400 mg, three times a day, 5-day course, *no alcohol*

Amoxycillin (broad spectrum—useful for general odontogenic infections)

    500 mg, three times a day, 5-day course

If allergic to penicillin:

either

Clindamycin

    300 mg, four times a day, 5-day course

or

Erythromycin

    500 mg, four times a day, 5-day course

Box B3.2 Suggested antibiotic protocol for patients presenting with diffuse swelling, fever or malaise. Always refer to the BNF.

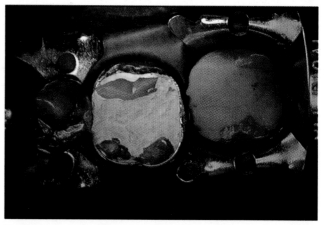

Fig. B3.23 Orthodontic bands may help to protect a tooth temporarily during root canal treatment.

Rubber dam

Rubber dam isolation is *essential* in endodontic treatment. There are no excuses to avoid using it. The main reasons for using rubber dam isolation are to:

◆ protect the airway from the risk of inhalation of endodontic instruments (files, burs);

◆ eliminate bacterial contamination of the tooth with saliva;

◆ prevent leakage of irrigants (household bleach) into the oral cavity;

◆ provide improved visibility for the operator by retraction of soft tissues (e.g. buccal mucosa and tongue);

◆ gain improved comfort for patient.

The essential kit (Fig. B3.24(a) and (b)) comprises:

▪ dam;

▪ dam punch;

▪ clamps;

▪ clamp forceps;

▪ frame

▪ dental floss tape.

Single tooth isolation

For the one-step technique, the criteria for success are:

◆ floss through adjacent contact points;

◆ select and try rubber dam *winged* or *wingless* clamp that gives four-point contact around the base of the tooth (Fig. B3.25a);

◆ apply gentle pressure with forefinger on bow of clamp to confirm that it is firm and does not rock;

◆ punch clean hole through centre of the rubber dam;

◆ stretch rubber dam over clamp and tooth;

◆ place napkin under rubber dam and apply frame;

For the two-step technique, the criteria for success are:

◆ floss through adjacent contact points;

◆ select and try rubber dam winged clamp that gives four-point contact around gingival margin of the tooth;

◆ apply pressure with forefinger on bow of clamp to confirm that it is firm and does not rock;

◆ remove clamp;

◆ punch clean hole through rubber dam;

◆ put rubber dam clamp on top of the rubber dam and push wings under the rubber sheet (Fig. B3.25b);

◆ place rubber dam and clamp with rubber dam forceps onto the tooth (Fig. B3.25c);

◆ slip the rubber dam under the wings of the clamp with a flat plastic (Fig. B3.25(d) and (e));

◆ place napkin under rubber dam and apply frame.

When a tooth is broken down extensively, there may not be sufficient sound tooth to retain a rubber dam clamp or the clamps available may not be suitably shaped to give a firm four-point contact around the tooth. In such situations, one or both neighbouring teeth should be included in the area to be isolated, in a technique known as the split dam technique (Fig. B3.26(a) and (b)).

Isolation of multiple teeth (split dam method)

The criteria for success are:

◆ floss through adjacent contact points;

◆ select and try a winged or wingless clamps that give four-point contact around gingival margin of the neighbouring teeth;

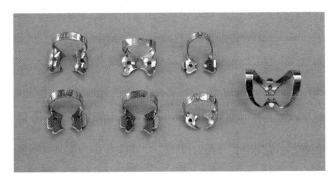

(a)

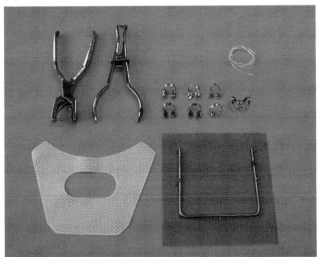

(b)

Fig. B3.24 Essential rubber dam kit: (a) rubber dam clamps; (b) punch, forceps, rubber sheet, frame, floss and napkin.

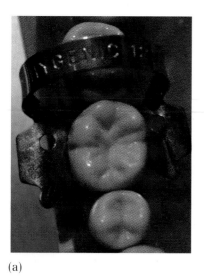

(a)

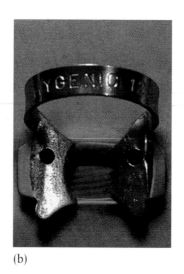

(b)

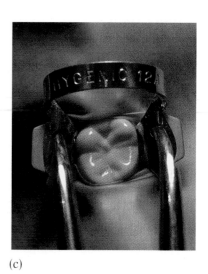

(c)

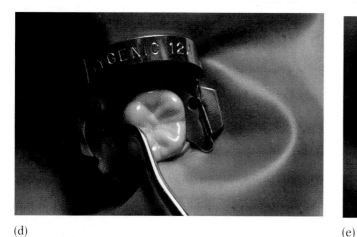

(d)

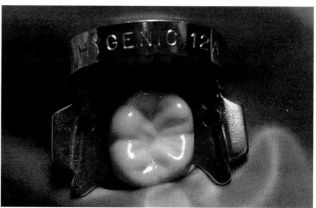

(e)

Fig. B3.25 **(a)** When trying a clamp ensure good four-point contact; **(b)** Securing the clamp to the rubber dam using the wings; **(c)** Placing clamp on the tooth using rubber dam clamp forceps; **(d)** Flicking the rubber dam off the clamp wings using a flat plastic; **(e)** the rubber dam secured in position.

- apply pressure with forefinger on bow of clamp to confirm that it is firm and does not rock;
- punch two clean holes through rubber dam 5–7 mm apart depending on the size of the teeth to be isolated and link them up by splitting the rubber between the two punched holes with scissors;

- stretch rubber over clamp(s)/teeth;
- place napkin under rubber dam and apply frame.

Alternatively, once the rubber dam is in place, proximal contact points may be secured with tiny strips of rubber sheet, Wedgets® or wooden wedges. This method works well when several teeth are being isolated.

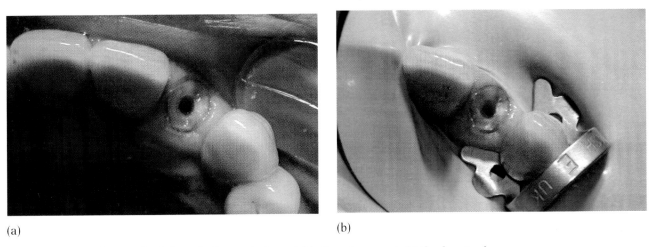

(a)   (b)

Fig. B3.26 Clinical example of the split dam technique: (a) before placement; (b) the dam in place.

If there are any signs of saliva leakage once the rubber dam is on the tooth (more likely with the split dam method) then caulking material (e.g. Oraseal® or Cavit®) should be used to seal avenues of leakage (Fig. B3.27).

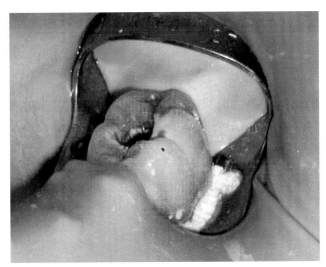

Fig. B3.27 The use of a sealing agent to prevent leakage around the rubber dam.

Preserving pulp vitality

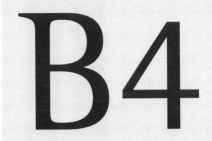

Preserving pulp vitality

Introduction

This chapter is concerned with those treatments (pulp therapies) provided to retain the vitality of pulps that are exposed (or nearly exposed). As explained in Chapter A2, a living pulp provides many benefits to a tooth, so it is essential to preserve vitality wherever possible.

Teeth affected by extensive caries are at risk of carious exposure during cavity preparation. Stepwise excavation is a technique that affords an opportunity for the deposition of tertiary dentine between visits, so allowing removal of all softened (and presumably infected) dentine. Techniques for direct pulp capping and pulpotomy are also suggested, together with criteria for the assessment of the outcome and prognosis of pulp therapy.

Stepwise excavation

The criteria for successful stepwise excavation are (Fig. B4.1):

- adequate local anaesthesia and isolation with rubber dam;
- excavate completely carious dentine at the amelo-dentinal junction;
- excavate remaining caries from the rest of the cavity, leaving only carious dentine directly overlying the pulp;
- place a calcium hydroxide lining in the deep areas of the cavity;
- restore the entire cavity (e.g. IRM®/glass-ionomer cement);
- 2+ months later isolate the tooth and remove the temporary restoration and lining material; if sufficient tertiary dentine has been laid down, excavation of remaining carious dentine will be possible without exposing the pulp;
- restore tooth definitively.

Note: at the 're-entry stage', if the dentine feels soft or a carious exposure occurs during final excavation then this is an indication to commence root canal treatment.

Direct pulp caps

The criteria for successful direct pulp capping are Fig. B4.2(a)–(b):

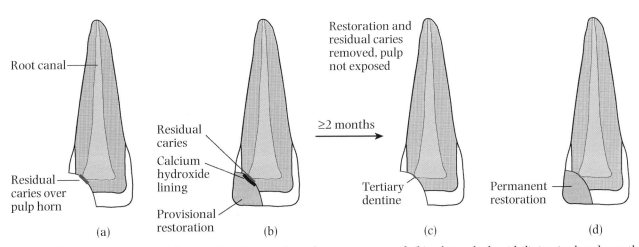

Fig. B4.1 Stepwise excavation: (a) caries directly over the pulp is not excavated; (b) calcium hydroxide lining is placed over the caries; (c) 2 months later the remaining caries can be excavated without exposing the pulp due to tertiary dentine deposition; (d) a permanent restoration is placed to restore the tooth.

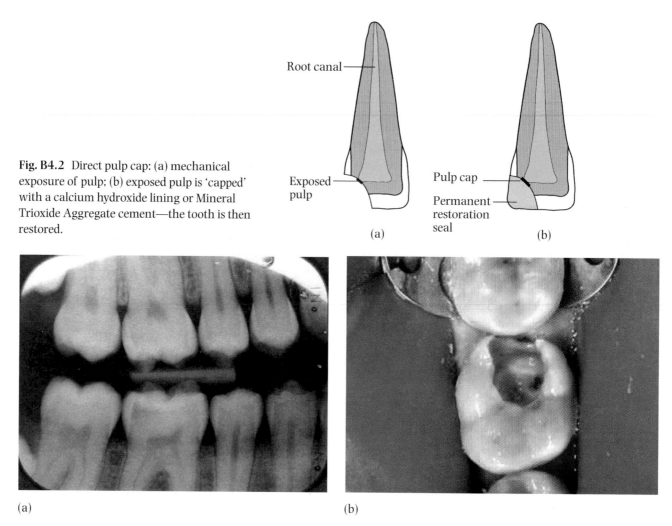

Fig. B4.2 Direct pulp cap: (a) mechanical exposure of pulp; (b) exposed pulp is 'capped' with a calcium hydroxide lining or Mineral Trioxide Aggregate cement—the tooth is then restored.

Root canal

Exposed pulp

Pulp cap

Permanent restoration seal

(a)

(b)

(a)

(b)

Fig. B4.3 (a) Bitewing radiograph of mandibular first molar showing extent of carious lesion; (b) exposed pulp isolated following removal of caries and rinsing with sodium hypochlorite.

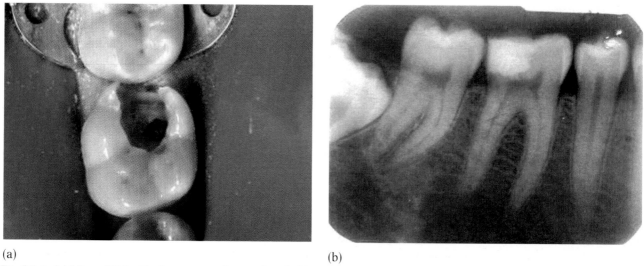

(a)

(b)

Fig. B4.4 (a) Mineral Trioxide Aggregate pulp cap placed; (b) Post-operative periapical radiograph following provisional restoration.

- adequate local anaesthesia and isolation with rubber dam (Fig. B4.3(a) & (b));

- carious lesion (if present) entirely removed;

- rinse exposed pulp with 0.5% sodium hypochlorite

- any bleeding of the pulp should stop after 1–2 min; if necessary, use a moist sterile cotton pledget to gently blot;

- apply pulp capping material (Fig. B4.4(a) and (b));

- restore tooth with a well-adapted plastic restoration (e.g. glass-ionomer base and composite restoration).

Persistent or excessive bleeding is a sign that the pulp wound is inflamed and is an indication to either perform a pulpotomy procedure or root canal treatment (Fig. B4.5). The prognosis of this procedure is adversely affected if the blood clot is not removed prior to application of the pulp capping material. The size of the exposure does not influence the prognosis.

Pulpotomy

The criteria for successful pulpotomy are (Fig. B4.6(a)–(b)):

- adequate local anaesthesia and isolation with rubber dam;

- rinse the exposed pulp with 0.5% sodium hypochlorite, then rinse with sterile, isotonic saline;

- amputate pulp in 1–2 mm increments until excessive bleeding stops (i.e. indicating that the inflamed portion has been removed); blood is removed gently by irrigating with sterile saline and the pulp stump is blotted gently with a moist, sterile cotton pledget; once haemo-

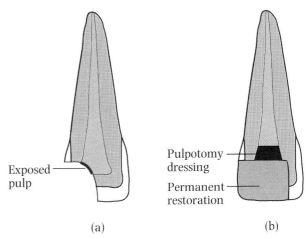

Fig. B4.6 Pulpotomy: (a) traumatic pulp exposure; (b) 2–3 mm of pulp tissue amputated with long tapered bur, a calcium hydroxide lining or Mineral Trioxide Aggregate cement placed over exposed pulp. The tooth is then permanently restored.

stasis is achieved the pulp capping material may be placed (Fig. B4.7(a)–(d));

- 2–3 mm thickness of pulp capping material is placed over the pulp and this is sealed in place with an antibacterial base (IRM®), after which the tooth is permanently restored.

The pulp is best amputated using a long tapered diamond bur with copious water coolant. To prevent tearing and additional trauma to the already distressed pulp, manual excavation and slow speed burs should be avoided; for the same reason cotton pledgets should never be dry.

Criteria for evaluating outcome of pulp preservation treatment

Symptoms

The patient should have no symptoms of pulpitis or periradicular periodontitis if treatment has been successful.

Clinical signs

There should be a normal, positive response to vitality testing, with no tenderness to percussion if success has been achieved. The tooth becoming discoloured or nonvital may indicate treatment failure. Periradicular involvement may be indicated by tenderness to palpation, tenderness to percussion, the presence of a sinus or mobility. Evaluation of the probing profile revealing a sinus of endodontic origin or discharging through the periodontal ligament indicates failure.

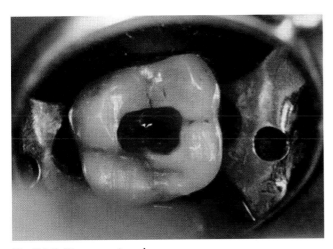

Fig. B4.5 Hyperaemic pulp.

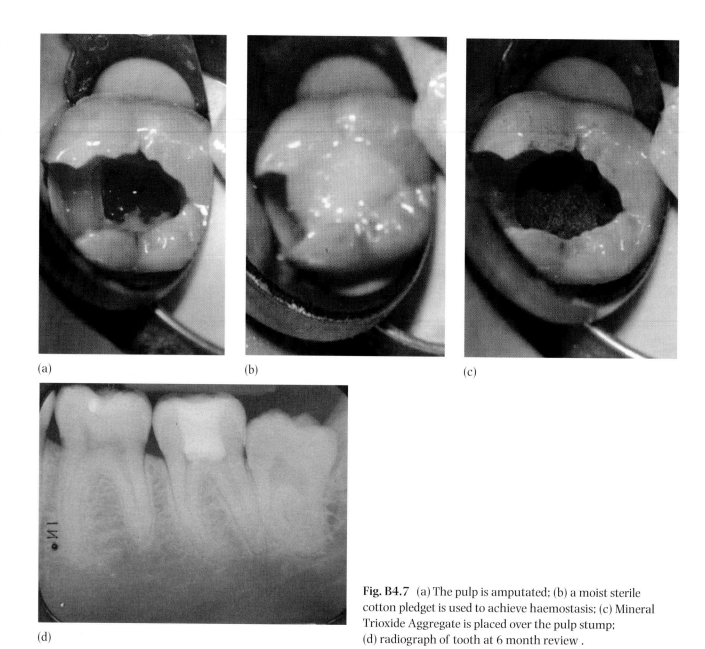

(a) (b) (c)

(d)

Fig. B4.7 (a) The pulp is amputated; (b) a moist sterile cotton pledget is used to achieve haemostasis; (c) Mineral Trioxide Aggregate is placed over the pulp stump; (d) radiograph of tooth at 6 month review .

Coronal seal

The quality of the coronal seal must be adequate to prevent contamination of the previously treated area.

Radiographic signs

In immature teeth there should be signs of further development of the root (compare to the neighbouring and contralateral teeth). The presence of a 'dentine bridge' (seen radiographically) at the interface between the pulp wound and capping material indicates a response of a vital, healthy pulp (Fig. A4.4(a) and (b)). There should be no signs of periodontal ligament widening or the development of a periradicular radiolucency.

As with all endodontic treatments, these teeth should be followed up regularly. When assessing the outcome of treatment, you are trying to assess if the tooth is still vital.

Prognosis

Pulp preservation procedures can have a high success rate providing the following criteria are met:

- Healthy pulp: The pulp is not irreversibly inflamed.

- Aseptic technique: Treatment is carried out under rubber dam to prevent the inflamed, but uninfected exposed pulpal wound becoming contaminated with microorganisms.

- Haemmorhage control: It is essential to remove any blood clot which will otherwise prevent adequate contact of pulp-capping material to pulp tissue

- Coronal seal: The pulp preservation site is sealed with a bacterial-tight restoration.

Root canal preparation

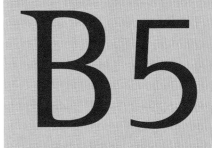

Root canal preparation

Introduction

This chapter discusses approaches to root canal preparation. There will be variation in the emphasis placed on particular procedures and practices in individual schools, but it is hoped that the *principles* behind most current preparation techniques are common, so confusion should be minimized. Root canal treatment should only be carried out once a correct diagnosis has been made (see Chapter B3).

Pre-operative radiographs

A periapical film of the appropriate tooth should always be available. The criteria for success are as follows:

- use a paralleling radiographic technique (Fig. B5.1);
- the complete tooth should be visible, including 3+ mm of periapical bone;
- create minimal geometric distortion (elongation or foreshortening of image) by bending of the film or errors of patient or tube positioning;
- employ correct procedures for exposure, developing, mounting and labelling of radiographs;
- assess for the presence or absence of a pulp chamber, its depth from the occlusal surface and the presence or absence of pulpal horns.

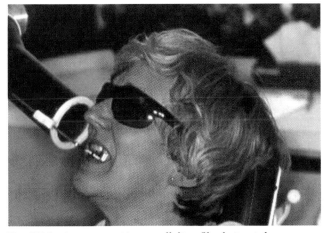

Fig. B5.1 A pre-operative paralleling film being taken.

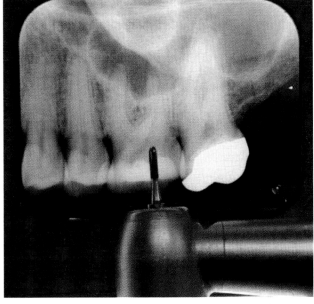

Fig. B5.2 A bur used to estimate the depth of the pulp chamber in a molar tooth.

Placing a bur (mounted in a handpiece) against the pre-operative radiograph is a useful method of estimating how deep the floor of the pulp chamber is likely to be. If the floor of the pulp chamber is obscured (for example, by the presence of a metal crown), the furcation may be used as a reference point (Fig. B5.2).

Access cavity preparation

The shape of access cavity to be prepared varies according to tooth type, arch and number of canals that are expected to be found (see Fig. A5.3). The pre-operative radiograph of the tooth should be studied (along with any relevant bitewing radiographs). These aid in assessing the position, size and shape of the pulp chamber. The nature of the pulp chamber and possible difficulties relating to it should be noted. These may include pulp stones, very shallow pulp chambers and the absence of pulp horns.

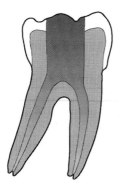

Fig. B5.3 Ideal access cavity preparation.

The criteria for successful access cavity preparation are as follows:

* remove the entire roof of the pulp chamber so that all coronal pulp tissue may be eliminated (note: anterior teeth do not have a pulpal floor—the pulp chamber merges into the root canal) (Fig. B5.3);

* produce a smooth-walled preparation with no overhangs of dentine (Fig. B5.4);

* create no damage to the pulpal floor (Fig. B5.5);

* allow unimpeded, straight-line access of instruments to the apical region of canal(s) (Figs B5.6 and B5.7);

* allow visualization of canal orifices (Fig. B5.8);

* allow retention of a temporary restoration;

* be as conservative as possible whilst fulfilling the steps listed above.

The bur of choice is a tungsten carbide cross-cut bur in a high speed handpiece for initial access preparation, followed by a non-end-cutting bur once the roof of the pulp chamber has been accessed (Figs B5.9–B5.11). Note that

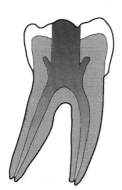

Fig. B5.4 Incomplete removal of the roof of the pulp chamber and overhanging dentine.

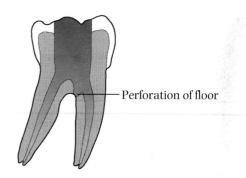

Perforation of floor

Fig. B5.5 Perforation of pulpal floor.

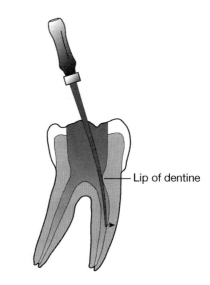

Lip of dentine

Fig. B5.6 Inadequate straight line access resulting in the tip of the file attemting to straighten itself – see arrows.

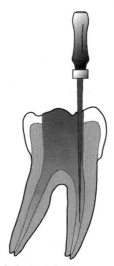

Fig. B5.7 Unimpeded, straight-line access to the root canal.

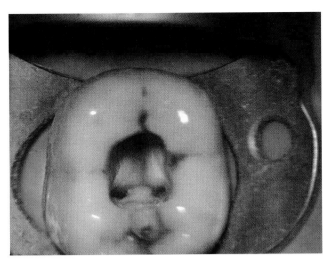

Fig. B5.8 Access cavity allowing visualization of the root canals.

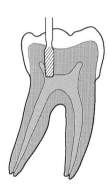

Fig. B5.9 Tungsten carbide bur penetrating the roof of the pulp chamber.

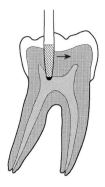

Fig. B5.10 Endo-Z bur removing the remainder of the roof of the pulp chamber.

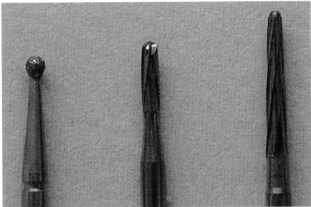

Fig. B5.11 Close-up view of burs commonly used in access cavity preparation. Left to right: diamond bur (accessing through porcelain); tungsten carbide bur (penetrating the roof of the pulp chamber); Endo-Z bur (for removal of the entire roof of the pulp chamber).

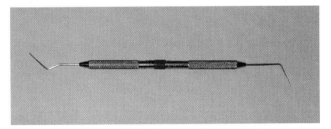

Fig. B5.12 DG16 probe for location of root canals.

porcelain cuts more easily with diamond burs, so if the access has to be made through a metal-ceramic or ceramic crown, a diamond bur should be used to cut through the porcelain.

Extensively broken down or carious teeth should be restored with a plastic restoration prior to preparing the access cavity, thus allowing easy placement of a rubber dam clamp and also creating a reservoir in the pulp chamber for irrigant.

The roof of the pulp chamber is penetrated through the central portion of the crown of the tooth as this is usually the region where the roof and the floor of the pulp chamber are at their furthest distance apart. When there is a space between the roof and the floor, the bur is felt to suddenly drop into the pulp chamber. At that point, the bur should be changed to a non-end-cutting variety (e.g. Endo-Z bur), the blunt end of which will prevent damage to the floor of the access cavity as the bur cuts away the roof of the pulp chamber and refines the sides of the access cavity. The pre-operative view should give an indication of the depth and size of the pulp chamber.

There may be situations where the canal orifices are obstructed by pulp stones or dystrophic calcifications. The roof of the pulp chamber should be removed with care, after which, small excavators or endodontic ultrasonic tips may be used to loosen and remove these calcifications.

Canal orifice location

At this stage, a 'DG16' endodontic explorer may be used to probe the walls of the access cavity to ensure that there are no lips of the pulp chamber roof remaining. The 'DG16' (Fig. B5.12) is then used to locate the canal orifices and to confirm that straight-line access has been established.

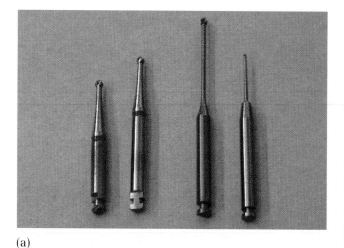

(a)

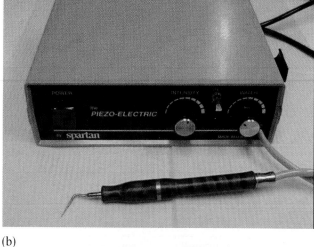

(b)

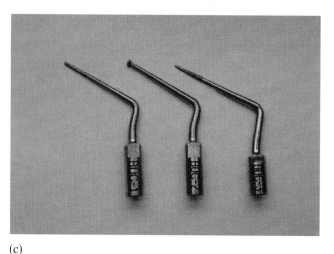

(c)

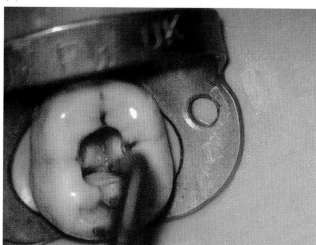

(d)

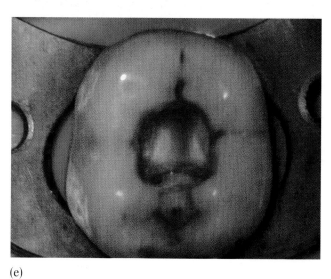

(e)

Fig. B5.13 (a) selection of burs used with a contra-lateral handpiece. Left to right: standard length rose head bur; longer shank rose head bur; goose head bur; Long neck (LN) bur (the last 2 burs have narrower shanks to improve vision). (b) Spartan ultrasonic unit and handpiece. (c) Selection of ultrasonic tips used with ultrasonic unit. (d) Ultrasonic tip removing tertiary dentine from the access cavity. (e) Completed access cavity preparation.

Removal of tertiary dentine

Excessive deposits of tertiary dentine may be removed gently with long-shank burs (Fig. B5.13a) in a slow hand- piece or by using ultrasonic units with special endodontic attachments (Fig. B5.13b–e), which are designed to remove dentine.

Pulp chambers may be partly occluded by tertiary den- tine and the canal orifices may be narrowed due to excess- ive deposition of tertiary dentine. In these circumstances, careful examination of the floor of the pulp chamber may reveal clues to the whereabouts of canal orifices. Secondary dentine is yellow and the floor and walls of the pulp cham- ber will be a similar colour or darker. Tertiary dentine in

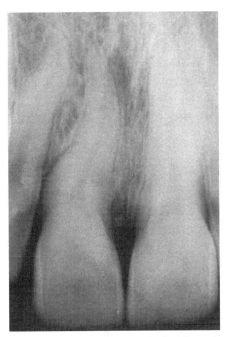

Fig. B5.14 Radiograph showing marked S-shaped curve canal anatomy in one plane only (mesio-distal). Are there any curves in the bucco-lingual plane?

contrast is more opaque and white. The use of magnification aids greatly the visualization of the access cavity and is highly recommended.

Coronal shaping and flaring

Once the orifice of a canal has been located, an undistorted size 8 or 10 file is used to explore the root canal to establish that the canal is negotiable. The ease with which this small file passes down the root canal may give an indication of the presence of curvatures that were not visible from the radiographic assessment (i.e. curvatures in the bucco-lingual plane) and also the joining or separation of root canals. Undue force may cause a blockage in the root canal and should not be attempted at any stage. These very small instruments should easily negotiate the root canal but lubrication (for example, Hibiscrub® or File-eze®) may be needed in narrow or tortuous canals to facilitate negotiation of the canal. The file should be carefully inspected on removal as it may reveal aspects of canal anatomy not fully evident on the pre-operative radiographs (e.g. curvatures in the bucco-lingual plane) (Fig. B5.14).

Prior to inserting any file into the canal system, an estimate of the working length should be made using the pre-operative radiograph holding a file against the film.

The criteria for successful coronal flaring are as follows (Fig. B5.15(a)–(d)):

◆ Instrument the coronal half to two-thirds of the canal to produce a gradual taper, widest at the canal orifice; use hand instruments (for example, size # 25–50 stainless steel instruments), automated instruments (for example, Gates–Glidden 2–4 burs or Ni-Ti orifice shapers), or a combination. Irrigate regularly with sodium hypochlorite;

◆ Use progressively larger to smaller size instruments as you move from the coronal to the apical aspect—each instrument creates space for the use of files of smaller size to advance further down the canal;

◆ If using Gates–Glidden burs, note that these can only be used in the straight part of a canal; the depth of penetration of the instrument being limited by the root canal curvature (nickel–titanium files, by contrast, are more flexible and can be used beyond a curvature);

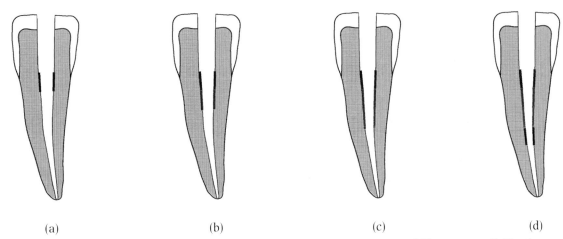

(a) (b) (c) (d)

Fig. B5.15 (a)-(d) Coronal flaring of the coronal two-thirds of the canal using a series of files or Gates Glidden burs, starting with larger sizes coronally and changing to progressing smaller sizes further down the root canal.

• At the end of coronal flaring the coronal half to two-thirds of the canal should have been prepared. The importance of regular, copious irrigation cannot be over-emphasized;

• Check regularly with a small size instrument (e.g. size 10 or 15) that the canal is patent (i.e. not blocked) beyond the level of instrumentation.

Working length determination

Once coronal flaring is complete, the working length of the root canal(s) should be estimated using measurements taken from pre-operative radiographs. The location and severity of curvatures should be noted, as they may influence the negotiation and preparation of the apical portion of the root canal. A common technique for determination of the working length involves the use of radiographs. The anatomical length of the tooth is measured using the pre-operative radiograph. An instrument is placed into the root canal to a length slightly shorter than this and then radiographed to confirm its position and determine the actual working length (Figs B5.16 and B5.17). An apex locator may be used to obtain a more accurate working length (see below).

Radiograph only technique

The criteria for successful working length determination using radiographs only:

• Refer to an accurate pre-operative radiograph;

• Estimate the canal length from the pre-operative film (described above);

• Identify a reproducible coronal reference point and ensure that rubber stoppers on the files are contacting a reference point before and after taking the radiograph;

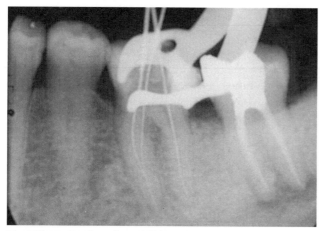

Fig. B5.16 Working length radiograph – note by the different instrument configuration that a Hedstrom File and a Flexofile have been used to distinguish the mesial canals.

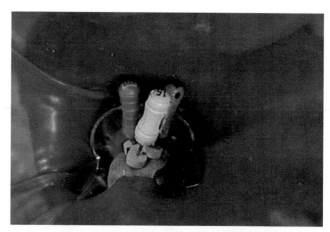

Fig. B5.17 Files placed in root canals for working length radiograph – note that the rubber stoppers are in contact with the cusp tips.

• Negotiate full length of canal using small files, with the aid of lubricant (for example, Hibiscrub® or File-eze®), if necessary;

• Use a minimum of a size # 10–15 file (smaller files may not be clearly visible, radiographically). If the canal is smaller than this, gentle instrumentation is required up to this size. In a large canal, use the first size that binds in the apical region. This is the *diagnostic file*;

• Take a paralleling radiograph of the canal(s) with file(s) in place;

• Aim for the working length to terminate at the apical constriction (the narrowest part of the canal). This ranges from 0.5 to 2 mm from the anatomical/radiographic apex *but* be aware that the discrepancy between the apex and apical constriction can be as much as 3 mm, especially in 'old' teeth;

• Annotate the patient's notes clearly, indicating the size of file used and the length from the coronal reference point; indicate that this is to be the working length.

Apex locator technique

Criteria for the successful use of an apex locator: See Fig. B5.18(a) and (b).

• Explain to the patient what you are about to do;

• Ensure there is no fluid (irrigant, blood or pus) in the pulp chamber or coronal half of the canal;

• Ensure the apex locator is switched on;

• Place mouth clip on patient's lower lip;

• Place a small file (for example, #10 or #15) in the canal and attach the apex locator clip to the file;

• 'Watch-wind' the file gently apically until the gauge reads '0' (the file is at the apical foramen);

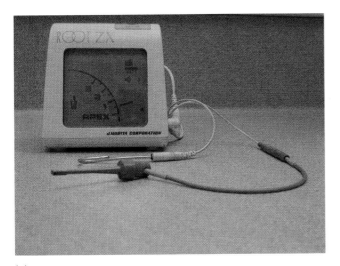

(a)

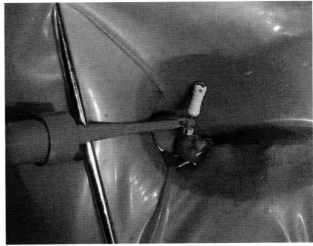

(b)

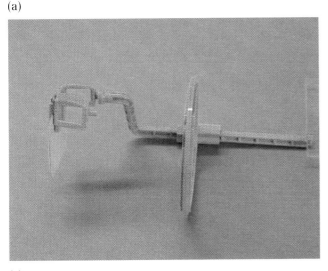

(c)

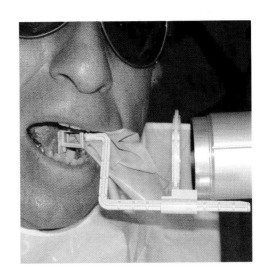

(d)

Fig. B5.18 (a) Root ZX® apex locator; (b) Apex locator terminal clipped onto file, the other terminal is hook-shaped and is attached into the mouth under the rubber dam. (c) Endoray® film packet holder designed for use in endodontics – the basket sits over the file(s) and rubber dam clamp. (d) Endoray® holder in use for working length radiograph.

- Ensure the rubber stopper at the coronal end of the file is contacting a cusp tip as this is the reference point for measurement;
- Remove the lip clip and file and measure the recorded length;
- Remember that the working length will be slightly shorter than this anatomical length;
- Take a diagnostic (working length) radiograph.

Working length radiograph

The criteria for successful radiographs are as follows:

- Employ a paralleling technique by using an 'Endoray' film holder (Fig. B5.18c and d);
- Position the file(s) correctly at the working length (or within 2 or 3 mm of the anatomical apex);
- Create minimal geometric distortion (elongation or foreshortening), by not bending the film or making errors of patient or tube positioning;
- Employ correct procedures for exposure and development;
- Visualize the complete tooth, including 3+ mm of periapical bone.

If the radiograph shows the file to be within 2 or 3 mm of that deemed to be the correct length, simple arithmetic adjustment can be applied if a paralleling technique has been used. Errors of a greater magnitude should be subject to exposure of a further film at the corrected working length.

If two canals are in the same plane (for example, bucco-lingual plane) they may be distinguished radiographically by using a file of a different configuration (for example, Hedstrom versus K-Flex files) in each of the canals that lie in the plane of the X-ray beam. The tube can also be angulated mesially or distally by 5–10° to 'separate' the canals (Fig. B5.16).

Apical canal preparation

Modified double flare technique

Once coronal flaring and working length determination have been completed, the apical third of the root canal can be prepared. This will be carried out in 2 stages: firstly, apical enlargement; and secondly, creation of an adequate apical taper. Once completed, the apical and coronal taper (*flares*) should create a uniform and smoothly tapered preparation. *Remember, irrigation must be used throughout all stages of preparation.*

The criteria for successful apical preparation are as follows (Fig. B5.19).

Apical enlargement

♦ Use files sequentially (small to large, i.e., #08 to 25) at the established working length, gradually increasing the size of the apical preparation;

♦ Start with the first file that binds at the working length;

♦ Irrigate between each instrument;

♦ Use at least two further sizes at the full working length, always checking the precise measurement of each file;

♦ The smallest acceptable apical preparation is usually equivalent to a size 25 (#25) instrument (though this may vary from school to school). The largest file that is used to the full working length is termed the *master apical file*.

The size of the master apical file (MAF) will be dependent on the curvature of the root canal and the original size of the canal. Therefore a central incisor in a young patient may have a #50 MAF where as a sclerosed curved mesio-buccal canal of a maxillary molar may have a #25 MAF.

Apical taper (or deep shaping)
See Fig. B5.20.

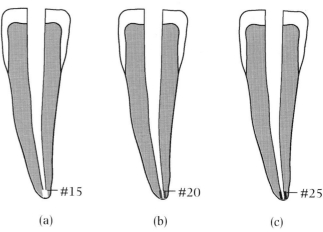

(a) (b) (c)

Fig. B5.19 (a-c) Apical enlargement from a size 15 up to a size 25 stainless steel file.

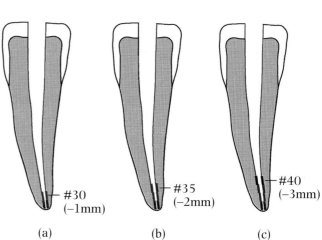

(a) (b) (c)

Fig. B5.20 (a–c) Apical taper created by stepping back in 1 mm increments.

- Use 3–4 sequentially larger files, each at a slightly shorter length (1 mm shorter than each previous file) to create a taper and blend the apical preparation with the coronal flare;
- Always use a gentle action;
- Irrigate between each instrument exchange;
- *Recapitulate* between each file size with the master apical file to the full working length, ensure the canal has not become blocked with debris;
- Create a smoothly tapered preparation, from entry into the canal to the apical constriction.

Apical–coronal approach (step-back technique)

With this technique, there was no early coronal flaring and all effort was expended on achieving apical preparation, followed by use of larger files at successively shorter lengths (hence, step-back). Gates–Glidden burs were used in the coronal third of canal preparation towards completion of the preparation phase.

This technique often resulted in apical compaction of debris, straightening of apical curvature and loss of length. It has now been superseded by variations on a crown-to-apex (coronal-apical) approach.

Coronal-apical approach (crown-down technique)

After coronal flaring and working length determination, the remainder of the canal is prepared (that is, tapered) by using files always in the sequence of larger to smaller sizes. Each successively smaller instrument will advance slightly further then the last instrument until the working length has been reached. Once the smallest instrument has reached the working length, the sequence is repeated with larger files until the desired file size is achieved at the working length.

It is important to understand the principles of what you are trying to achieve through canal preparation and it would be worthwhile at this point asking yourself whether you do.

Tips on preparing curved root canals

The creation of canal aberrations in curved canals (refer back to Chapter A5) when using stainless steel instruments may be reduced by:

- Using a coronal-apical preparation technique (e.g. modified double flare and crown-down techniques);
- Pre-curving instruments to match the curvature of the root canal;
- Using nickel-titanium (more flexible) instruments;
- Keeping the preparation small;

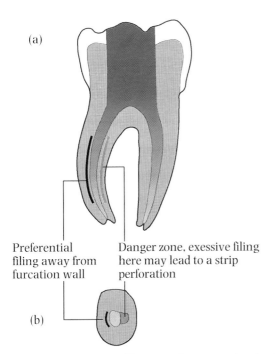

Fig. B5.21 Anti-curvature filing to reduce excessive dentine removal from the inner aspect of the canal. (a) Longitudinal view of tooth. (b) Cross-section of root.

Preferential filing away from furcation wall

Danger zone, exessive filing here may lead to a strip perforation

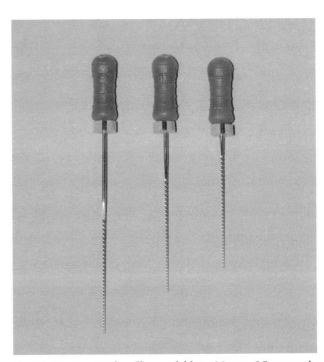

Fig. B5.22 Size 10 Flexofiles available in 31 mm, 25 mm and 21 mm lengths (left to right)— note that the cutting part of the file is 16 mm irrespective of the overall length of the file.

◆ Preferential filing of the outer walls of the canal, i.e. away from the furcation wall (anti-curvature), filing shown in Fig. B5.21.

Hand instrumentation

Stainless steel root canal preparation

The file size is based on the diameter at the tip of the instrument (see Chapter A5). Different sizes have an International Standards Organization (ISO) colour coding; it is worth learning. Each colour signifies a particular tip diameter. Hand instruments are also available in a variety of lengths (for example, 21 mm, 25 mm and 31 mm), although cutting blades are usually 16 mm in length, regardless of the actual length of the instrument (Fig. B5.22).

It is also worth developing an understanding of the mode of manufacture of the files you use, as this will have a bearing on the most efficient mode of manipulation. For example, the cross-sectional shape may vary and this will influence the flexibility of the instrument. The number of twists per unit length will also influence the flexibility of the files: the more twisted the file, the stiffer it becomes. The sharpness of its cutting blades and also the depth of the flutes between the blades will influence the cutting

efficiency of a file. Deeper flutes allow the accumulation of more dentine debris before the blades become ineffective.

Do not be lulled into a false sense of security that 'clever' files or gadgets are necessarily the key to success. The individual using them is a more important determinant.

Balanced force preparation technique

The balanced force preparation technique is described pictorially in Fig. B5.23(a)–(e). The principles are as follows:

◆ Use a clockwise quarter turn with gentle apical pressure to *engage* dentine in the flutes of the file;

◆ Follow this with an anti-clockwise half to three-quarter turn whilst maintaining firm apical pressure (the file wants to reverse its way out of the canal as it is rotated in this direction and you should resist this). This reverse turn *cuts* shards of dentine from the walls of the canal and a 'popping' sound may be heard as this occurs;

◆ Apply a further clockwise rotation through a quarter or half turn to *collect* the dentine debris on the flutes of the file;

◆ Remove the file from the canal and clean debris from it.

Further tips for effective use of the balanced force technique:

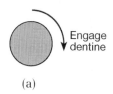 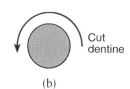 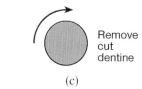

(a)

90° clockwise turn with *gentle pressure*.

(b)

180° anti-clockwise turn with *firm apical pressure*.

(c)

90° clockwise turn and withdraw the file.

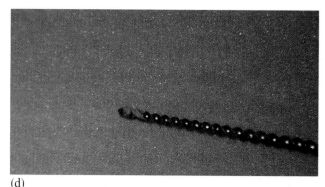

(d)

Dentine debris in flutes of flexofile.

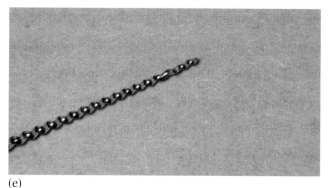

(e)

Distorted (untwisted) flexofile-further use of this instrument may result in separation within the root canal.

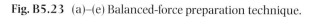

Fig. B5.23 (a)–(e) Balanced-force preparation technique.

- Repeat the first two steps a couple of times, then withdraw;

- Use this technique with stainless steel Flexofiles;

- Do not precurve files;

- Check very carefully for signs of distortion or unwinding of the instrument (Fig. B5.23e). Do not overuse any instrument and change to new files regularly;

- Ensure all debris has been removed from the file before it is re-inserted into the canal.

Here is a potentially confusing point: this approach works with stainless steel Flexofiles and hand Protaper (Nickel–Titanium) files, but if files of Greater Taper® are being used (Chapter A5), *reverse* the action (that is, turn in an anti-clockwise direction first) as these files are designed with the direction of 'wind' in a reverse direction to stainless steel. It is very confusing if you have been exposed to 'conventional' systems first. Note also that Greater Taper® and Protaper hand files can be used to refine preparations begun with stainless steel instruments or to prepare canals *de novo* using the crown-down technique described.

Automated preparation

Stainless steel and Ni-Ti instruments may be used in handpieces, this will be less tiring on the operator's fingers and also speeds up the preparation time.

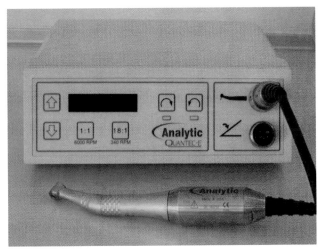

(a)

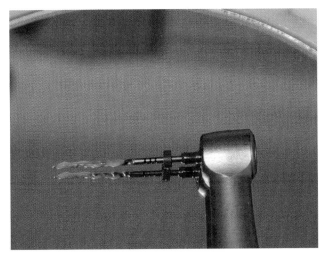

(b)

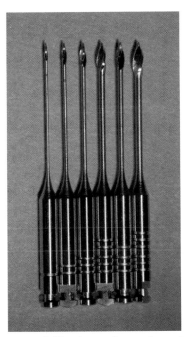

Fig. B5.24 Gates–Glidden bur—the mark on the shank indicates the size.

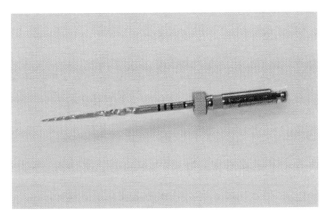

(c)

Fig. B5.25 (a) Electric motor and speed-reducing handpiece; (b) lubricant E. D. T. A. gel (Glyde®) placed on the file prior to inserting into canal; (c) excessive force and/or over use results in distortion of the Ni-Ti instruments.

- Use with a dedicated endodontic electric motor and speed-reducing handpiece (Fig. 5.25(a))

- Light touch required (the amount of pressure you would exert when writing with a lead pencil)

- Pecking motion—never force the instrument or keep at the same point within a canal

- The file must be rotating before entering and on removal from canal

- Use lubricant (reduces friction) and ensure that the pulp chamber is flooded with irrigant (Fig. 5.25(b))

- Clean flutes regularly

- Check files for signs of distortion before inserting them into the root canal and if distorted, discard (Fig. B.25(c))

- Monitor carefully the number of times (cases) for which files are used after autoclaving; if a canal system is moderately curved, dispose after single use

- Do not use in fine, sclerosed canals or those with severe curvatures

- Extensive practice on extracted teeth is mandatory prior to using on patients.

Box B5.1 Tips for using rotary Nickel-Titanium instruments.

Stainless steel

Gates–Glidden (stainless steel) burs may be used to prepare the coronal third of the root canal (Fig. B5.24). Due to their inflexibility they are limited to the straight portion of the canal. Six sizes are available: these are differentiated by the number of bands marked on the end of the instrument. Although these instruments have a non-cutting tip they may still remove excessive amounts of dentine and lead to strip perforations if used excessively. If the instruments break, this usually occurs at the neck, making them retrievable.

Nickel-Titanium

Nickel-Titanium instruments may be used to carry out the bulk of the preparation once the working length is determined and apical enlargement has been carried out to at least a size 20 stainless steel file. Ni-Ti instruments are used in a crown-down technique to prepare the coronal and mid third of the root canal. Before introducing Ni-Ti instruments into the apical third of the canal, the apical diameter has to be determined and a suitable apical taper has to be created with stainless steel instruments.

This process is known as *gauging*: stainless steel files are inserted passively into the root canal to determine the apical diameter of the canal and at least a size 20 stainless steel file should be used to the full working length. If the canal is narrow and/or curved resulting in the file stopping short of the working length, it may be necessary to carry out apical enlargement to ensure that at least a size 20 file does go to length. It is necessary to ensure that there is a suitable apical taper and this may be confirmed by *stepping back* 3 mm in 1 mm increments with sequentially larger stainless steel files.

Once the apical taper has been confirmed, Ni-Ti instrumentation may be completed until a suitably sized Ni-Ti instrument reaches the working length, i.e. an instrument with the same apical diameter as the largest stainless steel file which reached the working length in the gauging process. By following this sequence you will be less likely to separate instruments (Box B5.1).

Irrigation procedures

It is essential that the canal is irrigated at every stage of preparation with a bactericidal solution (sodium hypochlorite). The criteria for successful irrigation are as follows:

- ensure that rubber dam seals the working area;

- use a gauge 27 needle (equivalent to size # 40 ISO file) with Luer lock and cut-away tip (Fig. B5.26);

- only apply gentle pressure to the syringe to avoid irrigant being forced apically into the periradicular tissues (Fig. B5.27);

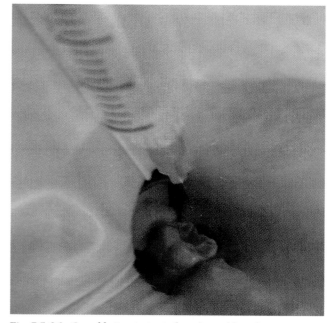

Fig. B5.26 Canal being irrigated under rubber dam.

- deliver in large volume and frequently throughout preparation of the access cavity and canal system;
- use 0.5–3.0% sodium hypochlorite;
- encourage irrigant exchange by alternating use with instruments.

With gentle use, irrigants are only delivered to the level reached by the needle in the root canal. This is usually at least 5 mm short of the working length. Therefore, it is essential to agitate and circulate the irrigant into the apical portion of the canal by recapitulating each time fresh irrigant is introduced into the root canal. In cases where the canal appears wide enough (for example, a maxillary central incisor) for the needle to reach the working length it should be premeasured to at least 2 mm short of the working length. Using ultrasonic instrumentation in conjunction with the irrigant may also aid its penetration into isthmuses and fins that are not readily accessible by instrumentation.

Smear layer removal

The smear layer may be removed by using ethylene diamine tetra-acetic acid (EDTA) as an irrigant, which chelates and removes the mineralized inorganic component of the dentine. Its effects are self-limiting and it has been suggested that it can be used in alternation with sodium hypochlorite. Both irrigants will flush out debris; sodium hypochlorite will also dissolve organic tissue (collagen) and is antibacterial, whilst EDTA will dissolve the inorganic component (hydroxyapatite) of the dentine (Fig. B5.28).

Irrigation in re-treatment cases

The use of chlorhexidine gluconate (Corsodyl®) or a solution of iodine potassium iodide (Betadine®) is recommended in the irrigation protocol of retreatment cases. It is suggested that a commonly infecting agent in these

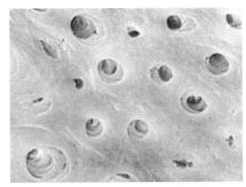

Fig. B5.28 Scanning electron micrograph of dentine following smear layer removal, note the 'clean' root canal surface and exposed dentine tubules.

cases, *Enterococcus faecalis*, may be resistant to the action of sodium hypochlorite. However, sodium hypochlorite should not be abandoned in these cases. Iodine potassium iodide may be used at the end of preparation, leaving it in the canal for 8–10 minutes before flushing out with sodium hypochlorite.

Placement of intra-canal medicaments

Root canals are dried with paper points to remove the bulk of the irrigant prior to placement of an intracanal medica-

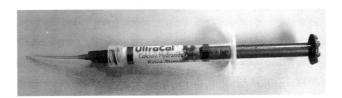

(a)

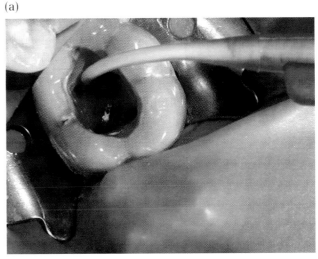

(b)

Fig. B5.29 (a) Syringe containing calcium hydroxide; (b) calcium hydroxide dressing being placed in a canal using a fine plastic nozzle.

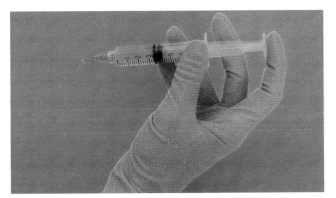

Fig. B5.27 Irrigating syringe – note that a forefinger rather than a thumb should be used on the plunger as this will result in the irrigant being expressed with less force.

ment, facilitating a greater volume and increased depth of placement of the intracanal medicament.

The criteria for successful intracanal medication are as follows:

- use sequentially larger to smaller paper points to dry the root canal(s);
- mix/place medicament onto a mixing pad (if using powder and distilled water);
- place the medicament deeply into the canal(s) using pre-measured #10 files or a spiral filler. Alternatively, it may be inserted into the canal using a syringe of calcium hydroxide with a fine plastic nozzle (Fig. B5.29 (a) and (b)).

Criterion–based self–assessment

It may be interesting for you to apply the criteria generated here (or variations on these appropriate to your school) as you practise the techniques of root canal treatment. Please use the boxes presented below to develop your own methods of self-assessment of practical experience. You will see that some of them are already partially completed—but you can, of course, change these. The important thing to remember is that whatever criteria you agree to be appropriate, ask yourself (and others) how well you have achieved the desired outcome. You could apply a similar approach to other chapters in Section B. These are examples only.

Tooth: _____

Pre-operative radiograph
Criteria (from Section B or devised by your school):
-
- *list them here*
-

Acceptable	Not acceptable	If not acceptable, why?

Coronal access
Conservative criteria for acceptable access opening:
-
- *complete the criteria*
-

Acceptable	Not acceptable	If not acceptable, why?

Radicular access
- creates flare in coronal half–two-thirds, removing majority of canal debris
-
- *complete the criteria*

Acceptable	Not acceptable	If not acceptable, why?

Diagnostic radiograph
- paralleling technique
- apex +3 mm apical bone visualized
-
- *complete the criteria*

Acceptable	Not acceptable	If not acceptable, why?

Preparation
-
- *complete the criteria*
-
-

Acceptable	Not acceptable	If not acceptable, why?

Irrigation
-
- *complete the criteria*
-
-

Acceptable	Not acceptable	If not acceptable, why?

Obturation of root canals

B6

Obturation of root canals

Introduction

This chapter provides criteria for successful obturation of prepared root canals principally by lateral compaction (condensation). It should be remembered that the qualtity of obturation can only be as good as the preparation will allow. The importance of the coronal seal is discussed again towards the end of the chapter.

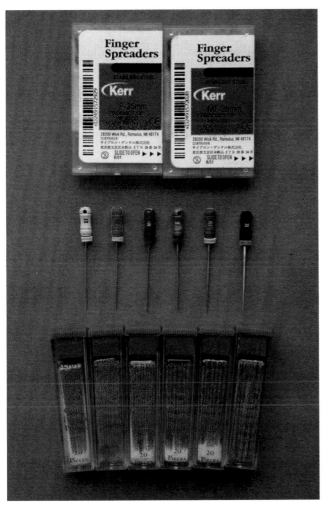

(a)

Which size gutta percha point should be used?

In simple terms, the *master point* for obturation should be matched to the master apical file size of apical preparation. If instrumentation has been carried out with instruments that have an increased taper (that is, nickel–titanium hand and rotary files), a point that matches the taper of preparation should be chosen as a starting point.

Lateral compaction (condensation)

The technique described here is widely taught and understood. It is simple, predictable and can be performed with the minimum of gadgetry.

Many of the newer techniques of obturation that have been developed (and may come to attract you!) are often dependent on expensive pieces of equipment and acquisition of particular skills. They do not necessarily produce better clinical results, though they may be quicker and in

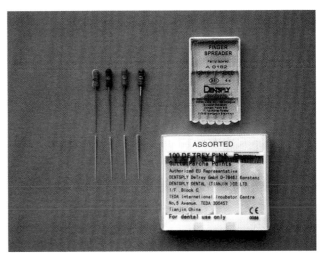

(b)

Fig. B6.1 (a) Kerr's finger spreaders and matching accessory gutta percha (GP) points; (b) Dentsply finger spreaders and matching GP points. Courtesy of Dr. M. Lessani.

experienced hands, less tiring to use (see the section 'common alternative obturation techniques' for a summary). The principle of lateral compaction is that lateral pressure applied with a spreader to a gutta percha (GP) point will create space for the placement of accessory GP points. The process is repeated until the canal is three-dimensionally obturated.

The criteria for successful obturation using lateral compaction (condensation)

♦ Select a finger spreader (Fig. B6.1(a) and (b)) that fits comfortably to within 1 mm of the working length. Finger spreaders come in four to six sizes (tapers) depending on the brand selected. Use a rubber stop to gauge its length, then remove the spreader and confirm its length.

♦ Select a master GP point that corresponds to the size of master apical file. Try this in a wet canal (this provides lubrication), using locking tweezers (Fig. B6.2). Feel for 'tugback'. Effective tugback is the resistance felt when the GP point binds in the apical region of the canal (Fig. B6.3).

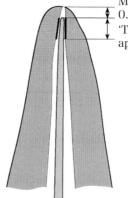

Master point should terminate 0.5–1mm short of full working length
'Tugback' should occur in the apical 2–3mm of the root canal

Fig. B6.3 The creation of 'tugback' of a gutta percha point in the apical region of a prepared canal.

Tugback occurring at a length short of the working length may indicate inappropriate master point selection (too large) or that further preparation is required. If tugback is absent, either select a larger master point or trim the tip of the existing point by 0.5 mm increments with a scalpel until tugback is achieved. (Alternative techniques are available to 'customize' the apical portion of the Master Point, for example, by dipping the tip in a solvent such as chloroform before trial placement, but this is tricky as the point must be very carefully repositioned in exactly the same way once root canal sealer is added.)

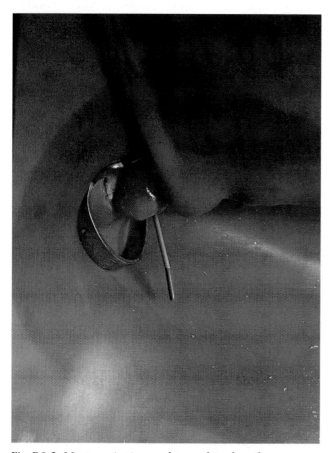

Fig. B6.2 Master point in canal to working length.

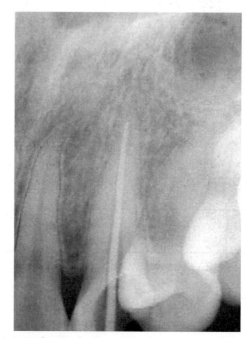

Fig. B6.4 Radiograph of trial master gutta percha point.

♦ Take a master point radiograph to confirm the length of the master point (Fig. B6.4).

♦ Successful master points should bind within 1 mm of the full working length with tugback—it is assumed that the pressure of lateral compaction will allow up to 1 mm of further apical movement.

- Dry the canal with paper points.

- Mix the sealer and apply it to the root canal wall using either a small file (i.e. size #10) or a small size paper point (Fig. B6.5). Apply the sealer to the apical third of the GP point and introduce gently but firmly to the working length.

- Insert the finger spreader alongside the GP point (Fig. B6.6). If the canal is curved, the spreader should be inserted along the convex (outermost) side of the

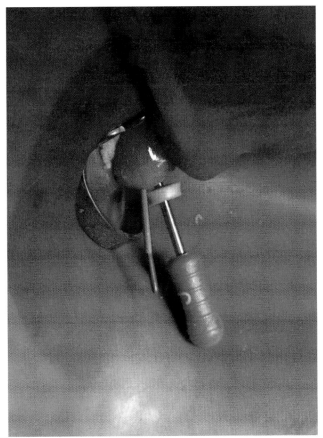

Fig. B6.6 Finger spreader placed in canal alongside master gutta percha point.

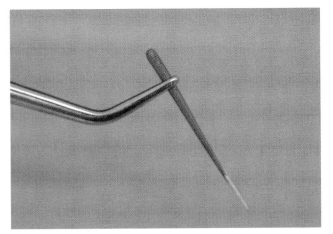

Fig. B6.5 Master gutta percha point coated in sealer cement.

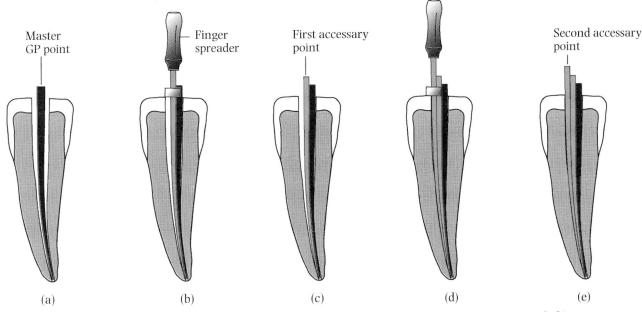

Fig. B6.7 Cold lateral compaction. (a) Master GP point lightly coated with sealer seated into the root canal; (b) Finger spreader inserted between outer aspect of curved canal and master GP point; (c) Accessory point cemented into space created by finger spreader; (d and e) Stages (b) and (c) are repeated until the finger spreader cannot create any more space in the mid third of the canal for insertion of accessory points. At this point, a mid-fill radiograph can be taken.

canal—this is less likely to result in the sharp tip of the spreader engaging the GP point and leading to the inadvertent removal of the point when the spreader is withdrawn (Fig. B6.7). Maintaining firm apical pressure on the finger spreader for 15 seconds will laterally and apically compact the GP.

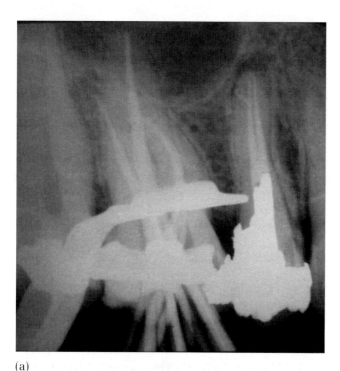

(a)

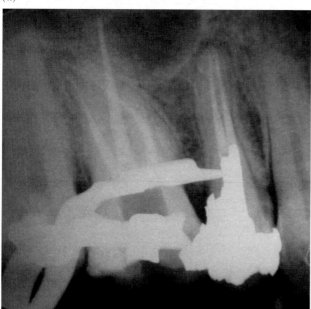

(b)

Fig. B6.8 (a) Mid-fill and (b) post-fill radiographs of molar tooth.

♦ Rotate the spreader clockwise and anticlockwise through 40° (or so), for several seconds whilst maintaining apical pressure before removing it.

♦ Insert a corresponding size accessory GP point in the space created by the finger spreader.

This accessory point should have a small amount of sealer placed on its apical 3–4 mm prior to insertion.

♦ Remove residual sealer from the finger spreader and insert it again into the canal as before followed by an accessory point until the canal is fully obturated.

♦ Take a paralleling radiographic view of the completed obturation phase. This should show a dense, uniformly radio-opaque mass within the root canal system, terminating at the apical extent of preparation. There should be no obvious voids in the apical and mid thirds of the root canal (Fig. B6.8(a) and (b)).

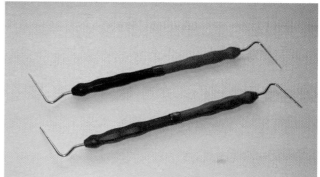

Fig. B6.9 Double ended Machtou endodontic pluggers for compacting GP.

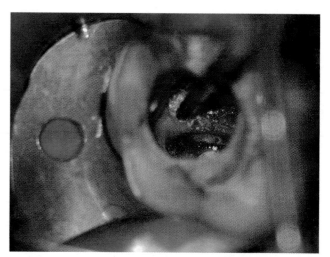

Fig. B6.10 Excess GP has been seared off with a heated plugger, and the remaining warm soft GP in the coronal third of the root canal is being compacted down with a Machtou plugger.

◆ Sear off the excess GP at the very base of the pulp chamber with a heated instrument and compact the coronal GP mass to below the level of the cemento-enamel junction/canal orifice using a plugger (for example, a Machtou plugger) (Fig. B6.9, B6.10).

The process can be modified (so-called 'warm' lateral compaction) where the spreader is heated, allowing easier compaction of the mass of GP and placement of additional accessory points.

◆ Place a base of glass ionomer or IRM® in the canal orifices and extend this over the floor of the pulp chamber (Fig. B6.11(a) and (b)). Restore the tooth, either temporarily at this stage or more definitively, if time permits (Fig. B6.12(a) and (b)).

Where two canals fuse, the canal which has been prepared to the full working length should be obturated first, after which the second canal may be obturated.

Common alternative obturation techniques

Two alternative obturation techniques that are popular with experienced practitioners rely on either warming the GP prior to inserting it into the prepared root canal (carrier-based systems), or warming the GP once it has been inserted into the canal (for example, vertical compaction). These obturation techniques should ideally be used in canals that have been prepared to a suitable taper with nickel–titanium files. Warming the GP softens it and

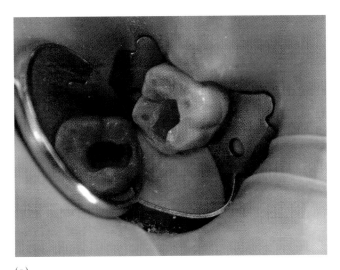
(a)

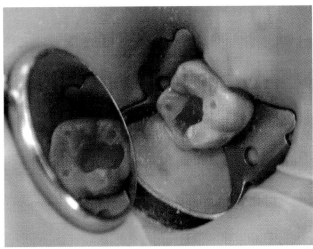
(b)

Fig. B6.11 (a) and (b) Glass ionomer placed over the canal orifices and floor of obturated pulp chamber.

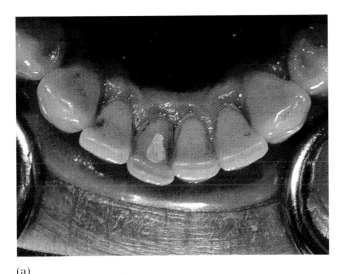
(a)

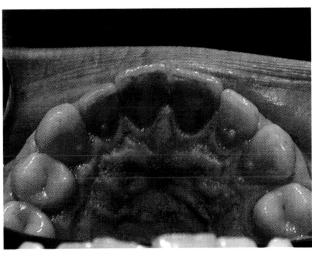
(b)

Fig. B6.12 **(a)** Temporary (IRM) and (b) definitive (glass-ionomer cement) coronal restorations.

this means it will flow more easily into the complex anatomy of the prepared root canal system, allowing easier compaction, resulting in a more dense root filling.

Carrier-based systems (e.g. Thermafil®)

In essence, a plastic carrier coated with GP is used to obturate the root canal (Fig. B6.13a). A 'verifier' (a carrier with no GP coating) is placed in the root canal to determine which size Thermafil® carrier is to be selected (Fig. B6.13b). The verifiers come in a series of sizes which have the same dimensions as the carrier.

The selected Thermafil® carrier is placed into a special oven to heat up the GP to a predetermined temperature (Fig. B6.13c). Once heated, the carrier is slowly inserted into the root canal, into which sealer has already been applied. As the GP cools it will tend to shrink slightly and pull away from the root canal walls, resulting in a poor quality seal. This can be counteracted by applying firm apical pressure on the GP for about 30 seconds. The handle of the carrier can then be cut off with a bur (Fig. B6.13d–f).

Vertical compaction (e.g. "continuous wave of condensation")

Once the root canal has been prepared, a non-standardized gutta percha point is selected which has the same taper as the master apical file. The tip of the gutta percha point is clipped with scissors or a scalpel until the gutta percha point is a snug fit at the pre-determined working length.

A pre-measured, electrically heated (System B®) plugger is then activated to vertically compact the gutta percha into the apical 5–6 mm of the canal. The taper in the apical third of the canal and the snug fit of the gutta percha point results in suitable resistance form to prevent the gutta percha from extruding through the apical foramen. Once the plugger reaches its pre-measured length (5–6 mm short of the working length), it is deactivated. Firm apical pressure is maintained with the plugger for 10 seconds to compensate for shrinkage as the gutta percha cools down. Then the plugger is activated for 1 second and removed from the canal. The GP from the coronal portion of the canal is removed from the plugger (Fig. B6.14a–i).

The mid and coronal thirds of the canal are then 'backfilled' with warm gutta percha expressed from an Obtura® gun (Fig. B6.15 a and b).

Open apex or blunderbuss roots

Immature teeth are difficult teeth to obturate. Often, there is no resistance to apical movement of GP points due to relatively parallel walls and lack of taper (a consequence of incomplete root formation). It is not the role of this book to discuss in any detail the management of complex situations and the interested reader is referred to advanced endodontic texts, although a glimpse of more complex obturation procedures might be of interest.

- Mineral Trioxide Aggregate (MTA) can be placed in the apical part of the root canal system using premeasured pluggers from an orthograde direction, resulting in a 3–5 mm MTA plug in the apical third of the root canal (Fig. B6.16).
- This is dressed with a moist cotton pellet to allow setting of the MTA.
- Access is regained at a subsequent visit when sealer and GP can be placed in the remaining space of the root canal. This may be carried out with a thermoplastic, warm GP injection system [for example, Obtura® II GP gun) (Fig. B6.15(a) and (b)] or by rolling several, large GP points together under a glass slab to produce a large point capable of achieving tugback.

Regardless of the obturation technique used, the end result should be the same (Fig. B6.17). The criteria for 'successful' root canal obturation (Fig. B6.18) are as follows:

- The entire working length should be obturated;
- There should be no voids within the root filling;
- There should be no overfilling (extrusion into the periradicular tissues).

It should be remembered that success in these factors is dependent on the efficacy of the preparation stage.

Coronal seal

As already stated, it is essential to place a coronal seal once the root canals have been obturated. A 2–3 mm glass ionomer cement or IRM® base should be placed over the obturated root canal orifices and pulpal floor (the majority of molar teeth have furcal communications with the periodontium). Restoration thereafter depends on the degree of coronal breakdown. Root-treated teeth appear to be more susceptible to fracture compared to healthy 'vital' teeth; this is mainly due to a combination of the following factors:

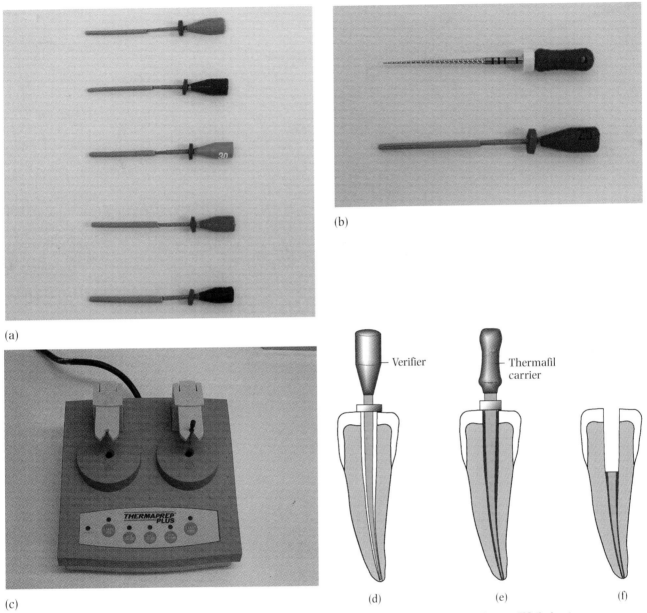

Fig. B6.13 (a) Assorted range of Thermafil® carriers; (b) Verifier (above) and equivalent size Thermafil® (below); (c) Thermaprep oven to heat Thermafil® carriers; (d) Verifier placed in canal; (e) Thermafil® inserted to full working length; (f) Handle of the carrier has been cut off and coronal GP compacted again.

- loss of tooth tissue (for example, loss of marginal ridges, remaining cusps walls are thinner and unsupported);
- loss of proprioception within the pulp–dentine complex;

Below are suggested guidelines for the restoration of root-filled teeth:

- A plastic restoration (composite restoration with a glass ionomer base) is indicated if the tooth (anterior or posterior) is intact apart from the access cavity alone;

- A plastic restoration may be adequate to restore an anterior tooth that has a small-to-moderate-sized proximal restoration. However, an extensively broken down anterior root-filled tooth may require a crown restoration;

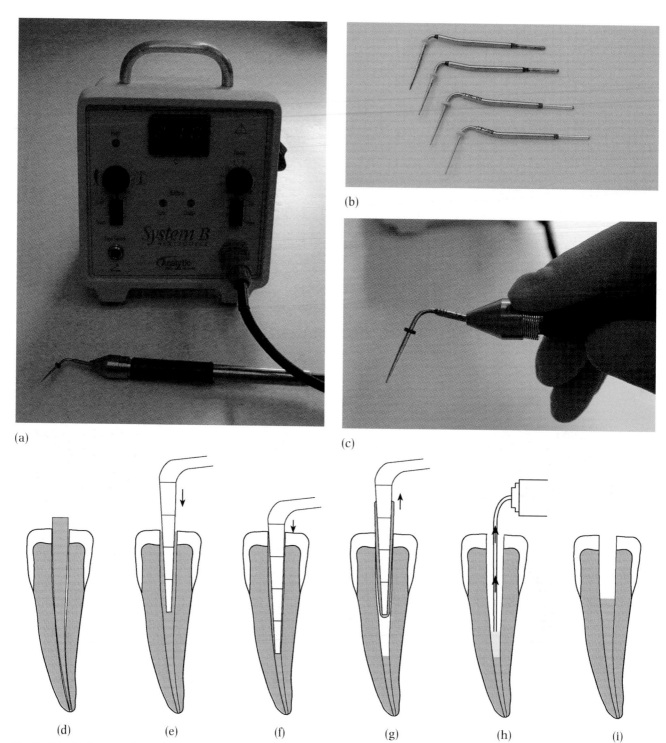

Fig. B6.14 (a) System B® battery operated unit and handpiece assembly; (b) System B® pluggers are available in 4 sizes and can be bent to follow the curvature of canals. The plugger which best matches the taper and size of the canal is selected; (c) The plugger is activated and de-activated by pressing and releasing the coil on the handpiece; (d) Non-standardized GP point cemented into canal; (e) An appropriate size plugger is activated and pushed down the root canal to its predetermined length; (f) Once at the predetermined length, the plugger is de-activated and firmly held against the apical GP to compensate for any shrinkage that may occur while the GP cools; (g) The system B tip is briefly activated to separate it (and the more coronal GP) from the apical plug of GP and the remaining apical GP is then compacted down with an endodontic plugger; (h) The remaining canal space is filled with GP from an Obtura® gun (see next figure); (i) The coronal GP is compacted with an appropriately sized endodontic plugger.

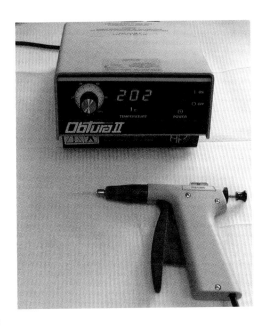

(a)

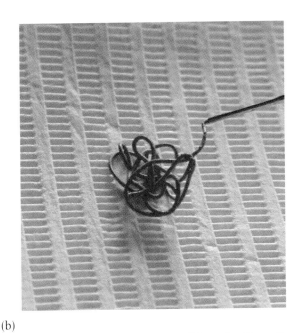

(b)

Fig. B6.15 (a) The Obtura® thermoplasticized gutta percha (GP) delivery system; (b) GP being expressed from the Obtura® gun.

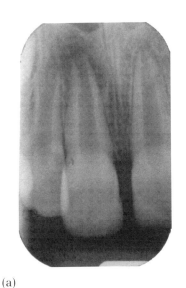

(a)

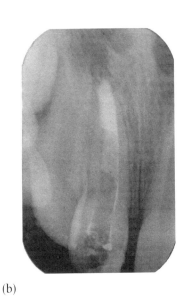

(b)

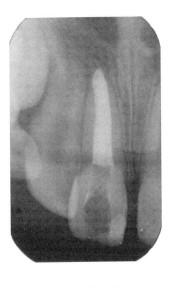

(c)

Fig. B6.16 (a)–(c) Radiograph of a Mineral Trioxide Aggregate plug at the apex of a young permanent tooth with an open apex. Courtesy of Mrs H. Pitt Ford.

- Root-treated posterior teeth that have lost one or both marginal ridges (Fig. B6.19(a)–(c)) require protection from occlusal forces, therefore consideration should be given to the provision of cuspal coverage cast restorations (for example, onlays or full coverage crowns);

- If there is insufficient sound coronal tooth tissue remaining to retain a core for subsequent crown preparation, a post may have to be used to retain the core (Fig. B6.20(a)–(c)). Do remember, however, that provision of a post, whilst providing (sometimes very necessary) core retention, does little for the health of

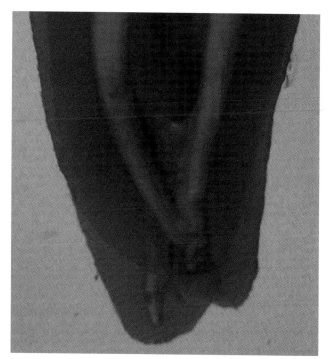

Fig. B6.17 A root filled, extracted molar tooth has been made transparent to demonstrate the quality of obturation that may be achieved. Note that the isthmus between the 2 mesial canals has been sealed with GP.

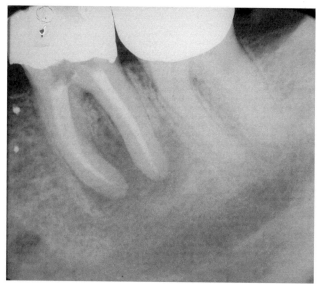

Fig. B6.18 Radiograph of a well obturated (and therefore well prepared) tooth. Note the uniform taper and absence of voids.

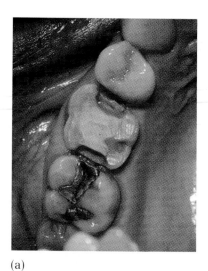

(a)

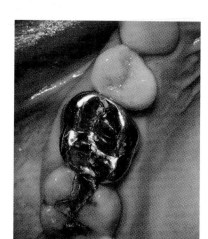

(b)

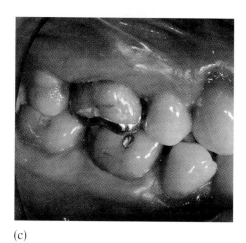

(c)

Fig. B6.19 (a)–(c) A conservative gold cast coronal restoration provides occlusal protection and a coronal seal for a root-filled maxillary molar.

the tooth as a functioning unit. It may weaken residual tooth structure and can lead to catastrophic fracture of the dentine, so the message must be one of the need to exercise great caution. A post is only advisable

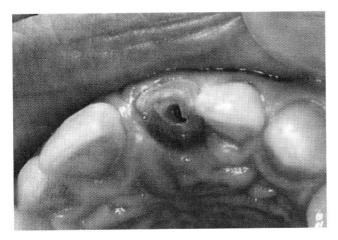

(a)

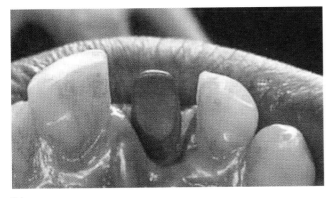

(b)

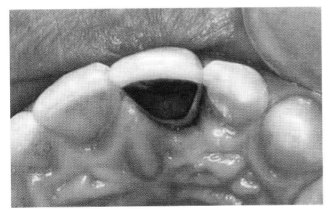

(c)

Fig. B6.20 (a) A root-filled anterior tooth where little coronal tissue remains; (b) a post-retained core is required to support the final restoration (c).

if no other restoration can provide satisfactory retention for the crown. One way of easing this decision-making process might be to make the necessary crown preparation before deciding whether a post is required. A decision could then be taken dependent upon the amount of coronal tissue remaining (in terms of available height, retention, and resistance).

Treatment outcomes

Treatment outcomes

How do we assess whether root canal treatment has been successful?

The technique to assess the outcome of treatment is similar to the protocol of clinical examination performed when a patient first presents with an endodontic problem. However, at this stage an objective comparison with the pre-treatment clinical examination notes may be carried out.

Root-treated teeth should be reviewed clinically and radiographically 1 year after treatment has been completed. At this review appointment the patient's symptoms, clinical and radiographic signs should be noted to assess the outcome of treatment. A note should be made of the stage of healing reached. Decisions should be made regarding the need for and timing of the next review appointment and whether further (remedial) treatment is required.

There are standardized guidelines published by the European Society for Endodontology indicating that clinical and radiographic follow-up should continue for 4 years. These guidelines should be endorsed.

Clinical findings

It should be noted that it is not possible to determine the outcome immediately after root canal treatment has been completed. This is due to the body's immunological response and whether there is evidence of apparent healing or disease as time elapses between completion of treatment and review.

A successful clinical examination will include an assessment of:

- patient's symptoms;
- tenderness to palpation of mucosa adjacent to tooth under examination;
- tenderness to percussion;
- changes in the periodontal profile;
- presence of a sinus;
- presence (and consistency) of any swelling;
- mobility;
- integrity of coronal restoration/signs of coronal leakage and avenues of infection.

The clinical findings should be noted and compared with the findings recorded before treatment was carried out, to establish if there has been any change. These findings should be recorded in a thorough, reproducible and objective manner to facilitate future comparisons.

Radiographic findings

The main points that should be noted from the review radiograph are:

- quality of obturation (Fig. B7.1);
- presence or absence of a periradicular radiolucency (Figs. B7.2a and B7.2b);
- comparison of size of the radiolucency to the pre-operative radiograph;

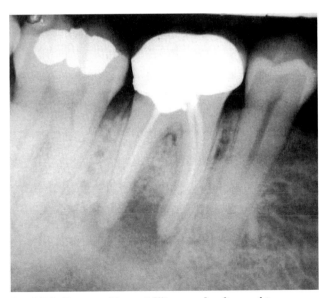

Fig. B7.1 Poor quality root fillings and radiographic evidence of coronal leakage.

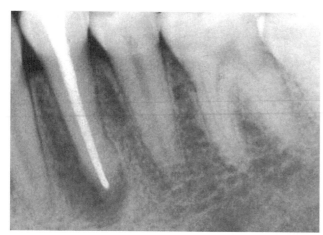

Fig. B7.2a Root-filled mandibular premolar with an obvious periradicular radiolucency at the time of obturation.

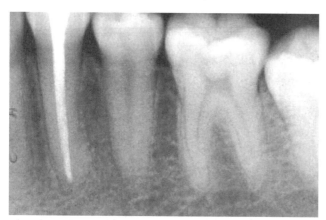

Fig. B7.2b Tooth showing an intact periodontal ligament space and lamina dura, indicating successful healing 1 year after treatment was completed.

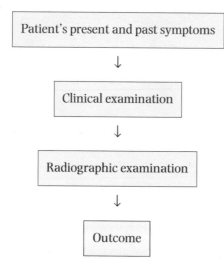

Fig. B7.3 Only after thorough assessment at the review appointment can a decision on the outcome of treatment be reached.

♦ avenues of re-infection, for example, caries or defective margins on restorations (see Figs A3.14(a) and (b) and A3.15).

At the review appointment, all the relevant findings are recorded and compared to pre-operative findings in a structured way.

How do we classify treatment outcome? (Fig. B7.3)

Criteria for successful healing

Clinical examination

♦ Absence of symptoms (or a significant improvement in symptoms);

♦ tooth in function;

♦ no abnormal signs (for example, tenderness to palpation or percussion, periodontal pocketing, sinus tracts, swelling and/or mobility).

Radiographic examination

♦ Radiographic evidence of complete bony infill in an area of previous radiolucency;

♦ intact lamina dura and an even periodontal ligament space (may be up to 2 mm wide adjacent to root filling material) (Fig. B7.2b).

Criteria for uncertain healing

In certain circumstances the outcome of treatment may not be so clear, resulting in the clinician being unable to categorize the treatment as a definite success or a clear failure.

Clinical examination

♦ Intermittent periods of slight discomfort;

♦ the patient actively avoids eating on this tooth;

♦ low-grade tenderness to percussion or palpation;

♦ tooth in function? (if not, through 'guarding' as opposed to a missing opposing tooth, this should be classified as a clear failure).

Radiographic examination

♦ No, or very slight, reduction of an existing periradicular radiolucent area/no positive radiographic signs of osseous infill (Fig. B7.4(a) and (b));

♦ widening of periodontal ligament space or loss of lamina dura.

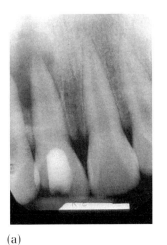
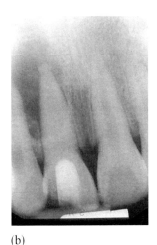

(a)   (b)

Fig. B7.4 (a) Central incisor with long-term calcium hydroxide dressing; (b) radiograph taken 1 year later showing no clear evidence of periradicular healing between assessments.

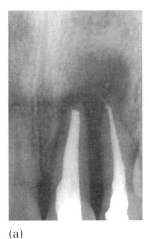
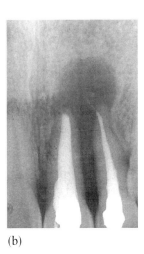

(a)   (b)

Fig. B7.5 (a) Incisors at the time of obturation; (b) a radiograph 18 months later, indicating a possible increase in size of periradicular radiolucency.

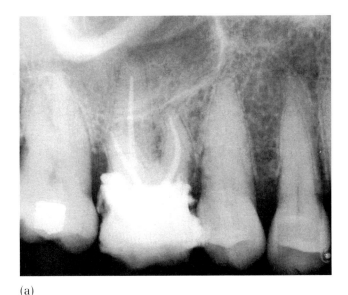
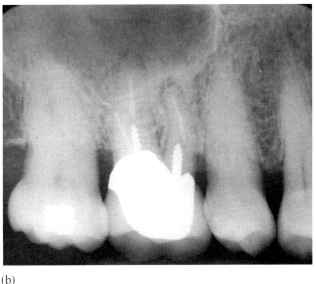

(a)   (b)

Fig. B7.6 (a) Maxillary molar at the time of root filling; (b) follow-up radiograph indicating widened periodontal ligament space and loss of lamina dura.

Criteria for failure

Treatment that has been unsuccessful is sometimes the easiest to categorize.

Clinical examination

- No change/no improvement/worsening in symptoms;
- recurrent or persistent sinus/swelling pain;
- no change or deterioration in clinical signs elicited (tenderness to percussion, mobility or periodontal profile);
- tooth not in function;
- avenues of re-infection (caries, coronal leakage, fractures, or periodontal pocketing to portal of entry).

Radiographic examination

- Increasing size of existing periradicular radiolucency (Fig. B7.5(a) and (b));
- increased width of periodontal ligament (more than 2 mm), loss of adjacent lamina dura (Fig. B7.6(a) and (b));
- newly developed radiolucency associated with root(s).

Dealing with failure

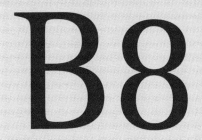

Dealing with failure

Introduction

This chapter is concerned with the practicalities of dealing with failure. If root canal treatments need to be revised, the coronal restorations on affected teeth may not facilitate access to the root canal system, so the first section of this chapter describes some methods to aid the dismantling of crowns. Removal of existing root filling materials forms the main section and the chapter concludes with a discussion of the principles of endodontic and corrective surgery.

Crown removal

A variety of crown-removing devices are available for use with single and multiple unit prostheses. Crown and bridge removers should be used with care. Tapping crowns and bridgework off with such instruments may lead to tooth or restoration fracture (Fig. B8.1).

Fixed restorations that are very retentive or have been cemented with bonding agents are likely to require

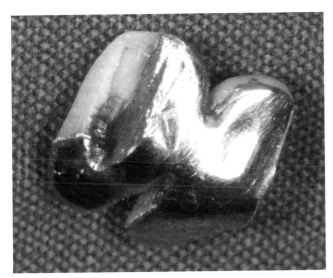

Fig. B8.1 Use of a crown and bridge remover has resulted in the fracture of the tooth as well as removed of the crown.

removal by sectioning. In this situation, burs should be chosen appropriately. Porcelain removal invites the use of diamonds whereas metal removal is achieved more efficiently using tungsten carbide burs, a point mentioned previously in Chapter B5.

Post removal

Most posts can be dislodged using ultrasonic vibration transmitted to the core through specially designed tips (Fig. B8.2(a) and (b)). There is a range of post-pulling devices that are used specifically for the removal of posts. These include the Eggler (Fig. B8.3) and Thomas post removal systems.

Removal of obturating materials

Techniques for the removal of GP involve the use of the following:

- Hedstrom files may be inserted around single GP points (Fig. B8.4(a) and (b)), then by braiding the files the GP can be grasped and removed from the root canal;

- Gates–Glidden burs or nickel-titanium files (Fig. B8.5) can be used to remove the coronal portion of the root filling. Their tips are non-end-cutting and frictional heat generated when they are used softens the GP;

- Gutta percha may also be softened by using a solvent (for example, chloroform) (Fig. B8.6). Solvents should be used with care as they will also soften and dissolve rubber dam;

- Heated instruments (e.g. old spreaders and System B® pluggers) and ultrasonically activated files may also be used to warm and penetrate GP.

The removal of solid cores (for example, silver and titanium points) and separated instruments may be achieved in a number of ways. Steiglitz forceps (Fig. B8.7) may be used to grip the end of the silver point. If it is impossible to grip the point, fine hand instruments may be passed between the point and the walls of the canal. By removing dentine

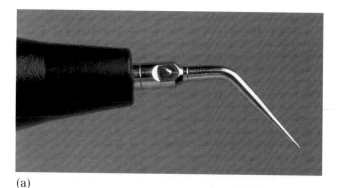

(a)

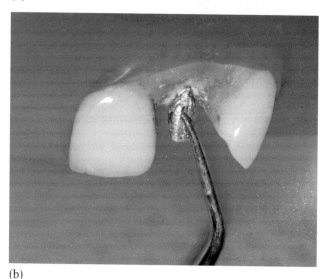

(b)

Fig. B8.2 (a) CT4 ultrasonic tip is ideal for post removal; (b) CT4 ultrasonic tip being used to remove a cast post-core restoration.

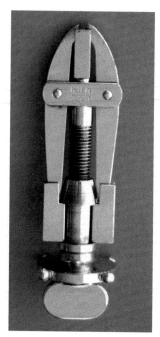

Fig. B8.3 Eggler post remover.

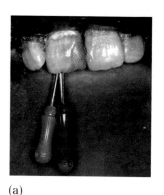

(a)

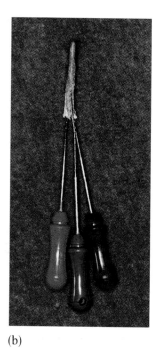

Fig. B8.4 (a) Three Hedstrom files used to engage a single GP point; (b) the GP point following removal.

(b)

from around the silver point, it may eventually be dislodged. Ultrasonically activated tips and files (Fig. B8.8). may also prove useful in a situation where a trough needs to be created around a silver point.

There is a kit specifically designed to remove silver points and fractured instruments. The Masserann Kit (Fig. B8.9(a)) consists of trepan burs (Fig. B8.9(b)) and extractor devices (Fig. B8.9(c)). The trepan burs are selected to have a slightly larger internal diameter than the obstruction and they are used to cut a trough around the obstruction to facilitate its removal. The extractor is essentially a rod that is screwed into a tube. The tube is placed over the fragment to be removed and the rod is screwed home to grip it (Fig. B.9(d)). The trepans tend to be quite fragile and need regular sharpening. The dentine so removed may also lead to weakening of the root.

Endodontic surgery

The scope of the surgical procedures used in endodontics includes incisional drainage, trephination, periapical curettage, apicectomy, root-end filling, replantation, tooth resection, root resection and biopsy.

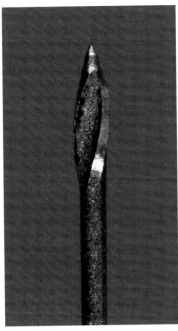

Fig. B8.5 Close up of the tip of a Gates–Glidden bur.

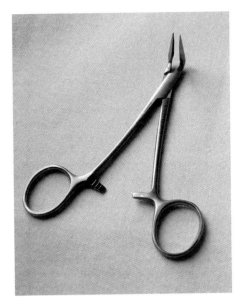

Fig. B8.7 Steiglitz forceps.

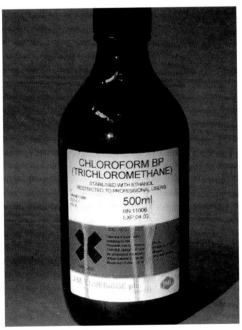

Fig. B8.6 Chloroform bottle.

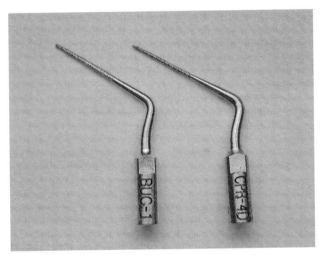

Fig. B8.8 Fine diamond coated ultrasonic tips are suitable for troughing around silver points.

Incisional drainage

When drainage through the root canal of a tooth is difficult, the incision of a fluctuant swelling (Fig. B8.10), to release the products of acute inflammation can relieve discomfort and bring infection under control as described in Chapters A2 and B3. In the absence of a fluctuant swelling, where infection is confined to cancellous bone, the process of trephination may be employed to drill and pierce the cortical bone to effect drainage. This can lead to damage of adjacent dental structures and should not be attempted by the inexperienced.

Apical surgery

This involves apical curettage, root-end preparation and root end filling procedures. Figure B8.11(a–c) shows a basic endodontic surgery kit.

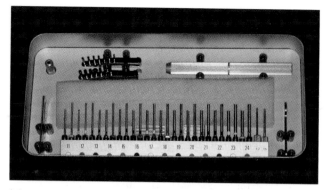

(a)

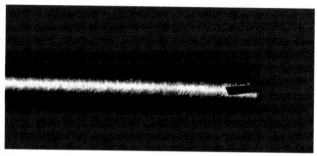

(b)

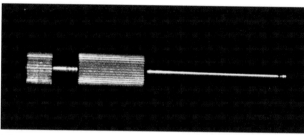

(c)

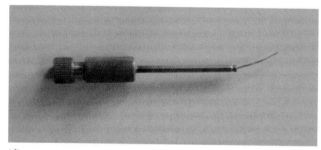

(d)

Fig. B8.9 (a) The Masserann Kit; (b) a trepan bur; (c) Masserann extractor, (d) silver point retrieved with a Masserann extractor.

Tissue flap reflection to provide vision and access is a fundamental consideration. There are many full and limited flap designs described according to their shapes and position. Flaps should consist of the full thickness of periosteum, mucosa, and gingival tissues. Flap reflection

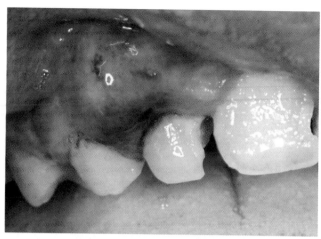

Fig. B8.10 A fluctuant intraoral swelling.

should be performed using appropriate elevators commencing away from the gingival margin. The flap should be lifted cleanly, separating the periosteum from the underlying bone. Once reflected, the tissue is held away from the surgical site by placing the retractor on bone to avoid tissue pinching. Regular irrigation of the surgical site prevents dehydration of the tissues. Location and identification of the root apex can be achieved using pre-operative radiographs, magnification, the presence of fenestration of the cortical bone and a sharp, straight probe.

Apical curettage involves the removal of a soft tissue lesion from around the root tip, before or after the apical portion of the root is resected. A root-end cavity is prepared using ultrasonic tips and finally sealed to prevent the egress of residual microorganisms and their products. Mineral Trioxide Aggregate (MTA) is the recommended material for this purpose (Fig. B8.12(a)–(d)).

Wound closure involves the placement of sutures. The sutured flap should be held under gentle pressure for 5–10 min before dismissing the patient with appropriate post-operative instructions. Sutures can be removed in 3–5 days. Residual scarring may arise in areas of sinus healing, relieving incisions and suture placement (Fig. B8.13) where surgical technique has been poor.

Success in apical surgery hinges on:

- good pre-operative planning;
- effective pain control and patient management;
- technical expertise.

Cases that need treatment of this type should ideally be referred to a specialist endodontist.

The following sections are provided for further information only. There is no suggestion that the dental student or recent

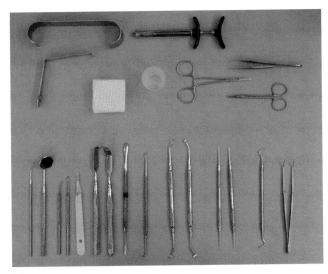

(a)

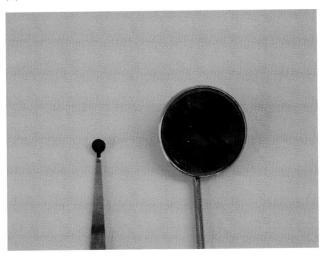

(b)

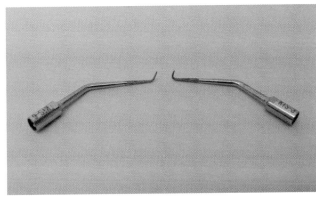

(c)

Fig. B8.11 (a) Endodontic micro-surgery kit;
(b) a micromirror (left) may be used to inspect the surface of
the root end; (c) surgical ultrasonic tips allow better access
and minimal preparation down the long axis of the root
canal.

*graduate would perform these techniques. It is important,
however, that you gain a working knowledge of the processes involved and cases that might indicate such treatment
measures.*

Corrective surgery

Corrective surgery is often performed to repair defects
in the root surface created iatrogenically (Fig. B8.14(a)
and (b)). These defects are referred to as perforations.
Traditionally, perforations were repaired using amalgam
and glass ionomer cement, but now MTA is increasingly
used for this purpose (Fig. B8.15).

Root resection

This term relates to the complete removal of a root from a
multi-rooted tooth without interfering with the crown
(Fig. B8.16). The indications for this procedure are periodontal disease, resorption, vertical fractures and failed
endodontic treatment that can be treated in no other
way than extraction. The procedure usually involves
flap reflection, resection, bone remodelling and tooth
contouring to assist with plaque control.

Tooth resection

Tooth resection is slightly different from root resection
in that it involves the cutting off of associated crown
material along with root substance. A portion of the
tooth is usually extracted and the remaining part is
restored (Fig. B8.17). Occasionally both parts are retained
and restored in a process often referred to as bicuspidization.

Replantation

Replantation may be performed intentionally in situations
where other surgical options are not indicated. In essence,
the tooth is extracted and modified out of the mouth in
such a way as to facilitate the disinfection and sealing of
the root canals. The tooth is returned to its socket and
splinted for less than a week. An example is given of a
mandibular premolar, which was extracted and replanted
to avoid apical surgery (Fig. B8.18).

Marsupialization and decompression

Large periradicular lesions may be treated by a surgical
technique that involves penetration of the lesion through
the cortical plate. Patency of the fistula is maintained
by the use of a drain or, preferably, a flanged cannula. The
marsupialized lesion may be irrigated and, with time,
the lesion reduces in size until the decompression can be
terminated.

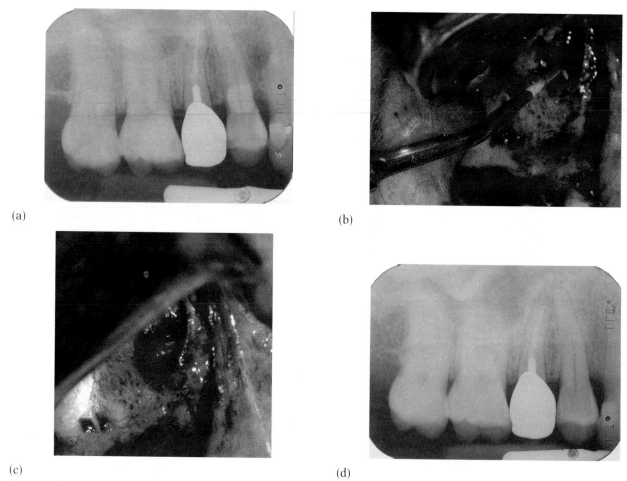

(a)

(b)

(c)

(d)

Fig. B8.12 (a) Failing root canal treatment: the existing post-crown is over 15 years old and has never de-cemented; (b) ultrasonic tip used to create a root end cavity (note how small the osteotomy site is after 3 mm of the root tip has been apicected; (c) MTA root end filling; (d) follow-up radiograph taken 1 year later shows signs of healing.

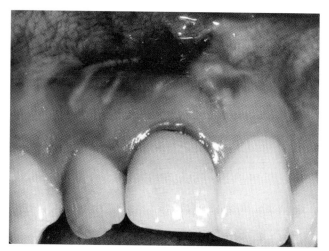

Fig. B8.13 Residual scarring in an area where endodontic surgery has occurred above an upper right central and lateral incisor.

Biopsy

Any tissue removed during surgery *must* be sent for routine histological examination to confirm the nature of the lesion. The sample should be forwarded for examination in 10% formalin and should be accompanied with comprehensive case details.

Conclusion

In some ways, it is unfortunate that this, the last chapter of the book has focused on the management of failure—as the purpose of writing the text, throughout, has been to attempt to demystify the principles of endodontics and thereby improve the probability of successful diagnosis

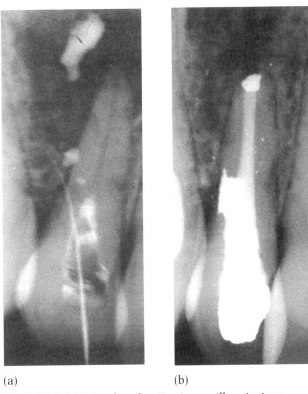

(a)   (b)

Fig. B8.14 (a) Lateral perforation in maxillary incisor; (b) radiograph taken following surgery and perforation repair.

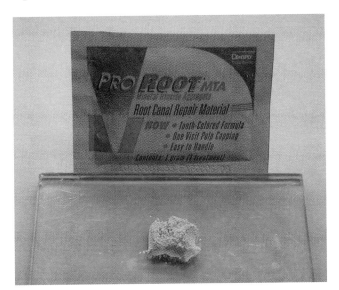

Fig. B8.15 Mineral Trioxide Aggregate.

and treatment. As stated at the beginning of Chapter A8, whist it is important to recognize that failure does sometimes occur, the challenge for us all is to learn from that failure—and to anticipate and strive to prevent its occurrence in the future through continued learning and the acquisition of new and enhanced skills.

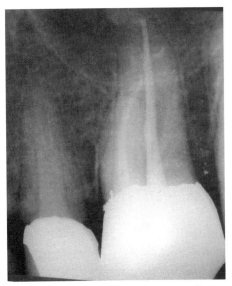

Fig. B8.16 Radiograph of maxillary molar following resection of the disto-buccal root.

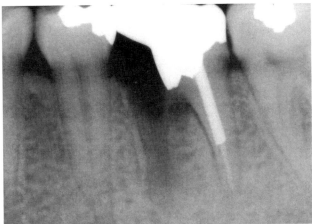

Fig. B8.17 Radiograph of resected and restored mandibular molar.

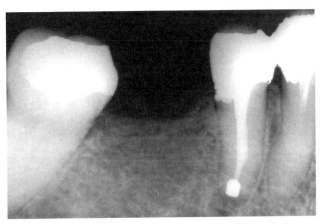

Fig. B8.18 Replanted mandibular premolar. The patient decided against endodontic surgery due to the close proximity of the mental foramen to the surgery site.

We have referred the reader to more 'standard' texts at various points in the book; it is hoped that your interest in this essential aspect of clinical dentistry may have been sparked and that deeper knowledge and understanding may be sought as a result, with the aim of increasing your enthusiasm and the quality of care that you provide for your patients.

Suggested further reading

Suggested further reading

1 Introduction

DE MOOR RJG, HOMMEZ GMG, DE BOEVER JG, MARTENS GEI, DELMÉ KIM (2000) Periapical health related to the quality of root canal treatment in a Belgian population. *International Endodontic Journal* 33, 113–120.

HOMMEZ GMG, COPPENS CRM, DE MOOR RJG (2002) Periapical health related to the quality of coronal restorations and root fillings. *International Endodontic Journal* 35, 680–689.

HUNTER W (1911) The role of sepsis and antisepsis in medicine. *Lancet* 1, 79–86.

KAKEHASHI S, STANLEY HR, FITZGERALD RJ (1965) The effects of surgical exposures of dental pulps in germ free and conventional laboratory rats. *Oral Surgery, Oral Medicine, Oral Pathology* 20, 340–349.

KIRKEVANG LL, HÖRSTED-BINDSLEV P, ØRSTAVIK D, WENZEL A (2001) Frequency and distribution of endodontically treated teeth and apical periodontitis in an urban Danish population. *International Endodontic Journal* 34, 198–205.

MARQUES MD, MOREIRA B, ERIKSEN HM (1998) Prevalence of apical periodontitis and results of endodontic treatment in an adult Portuguese population. *International Endodontic Journal* 31, 161–165.

MILLER WD (1894) An introduction to the study of the bacterio-pathology of the dental pulp. *Dental Cosmos* 36, 505–28.

MURRAY CA, SAUNDERS WP (2000) Root canal treatment and general health: a review of the literature. *International Endodontic Journal* 33, 1–18.

SAUNDERS WP, SAUNDERS EM, SADIQ J, CRUICKSHANK E (1997) Technical standard of root canal treatment in an adult Scottish population. *British Dental Journal* 183, 383–386.

SEYMOUR RA, STEELE JG (1997) Is there a link between periodontal disease and coronary heart disease? *British Dental Journal* 184, 33–38.

WEIGER R, HITZLER S, HERMLE G, LÖST C (1997) Periapical status, quality of root canal fillings and estimated endodontic treatment needs in an urban German population. *Endodontics and Dental Traumatology* 13, 69–74.

2 The life of a tooth

BRÄNNSTRÖM M (1986) The hydrodynamic theory of dentinal pain: sensation in preparations, caries and the dentinal crack syndrome. *Journal of Endodontics* 12, 453–457.

DAHLEN G, HAAPASALO M (1998) Microbiology of apical periodontitis. In: Ørstavik D, Pitt Ford TR, eds. *Essential Endodontology: prevention and treatment of apical periodontitis.* 1st edn. Oxford: Blackwell Science.

GENET JM, HART AAM, WESSELINK PR, THODEN VAN VELZEN (1987) Pre-operative and operative factors associated with pain after the first endodontic visit. *International endodontic Journal* 20, 53–64.

KAKEHASHI S, STANLEY HR, FITZGERALD RJ (1965) The effects of surgical exposures of dental pulps in germ-free and conventional laboratory rats. *Oral Surgery, Oral Medicine, Oral Pathology* 19, 91–96.

MORRANT GA (1977) Dental Instrumentation and pulpal injury. Part II clinical considerations. *Journal of the British Endodontic Society* 10, 55–63.

NAIR PNR (1997) Apical periodontitis: a dynamic encounter between root canal infection and host response. *Periodontology 2000* 13, 121–148.

TROPE M, SIGURDSSON A (1998) Clinical manifestations and diagnosis. In: Ørstavik D, Pitt Ford TR, eds. *Essential Endodontology. Prevention and treatment of apical periodontitis. 1st edn. pp 157–178.* Oxford, UK: Blackwell Science.

TROWBRIDGE H (1981) Pathogenesis of pulpitis resulting form dental caries. Journal of Endodontics 7, 52–60.

VAN HASSEL HJ (1971) Physiology of the human dental pulp. *Oral Surgery, Oral Medicine, Oral Pathology* 32, 126–134.

3 Diagnosis and treatment planning

ABOU-RASS M (1982) The stressed pulp condition: an endodontic-restorative diagnostic concept. *Journal of Prosthetic Dentistry* 48, 264–267.

BAKLAND LK, ANDREASEN JO (2004) Dental Traumatology: Essential diagnosis and treatment planning. *Endodontic Topics* 7, 14–34.

BENDER IB (1997) Factors influencing the radiographic appearance of bony lesions. *Journal of Endodontics* 23, 5–14.

ESCUDIER MP (2004) General and systemic aspects of endodontics. In: Pitt Ford TR, ed. *Harty's Endodontics in Clinical Practice.* 5th edn. London, Wright.

PITT FORD TR, RHODES JS, PITT FORD H (2002) History, diagnosis and treatment planning. In: Pitt Ford TR, Rhodes JS, Pitt Ford H. *Problem-solving in clinical practice.* 1st edn. London: Martin-Dunitz.

ROWE AHR, PITT FORD TR (1990) The assessment of pulpal vitality. *International Endodontic Journal* 23, 77–83.

TRONSTAD L (2003) Endodontic examination and diagnosis. In: Tronstad L, *Clinical Endodontics.* 2nd edn, Stuttgart, Thieme.

4 Preserving pulp vitality

COX CF, BERGENHOLTZ G, FITZGERALD M, HEYS DR, HEYS RJ, AVERY JK, BAKER JA (1982) Capping of the dental pulp mechanically exposed to the oral microflora-a 5-week observation of wound healing in the monkey. *Journal of Oral Pathology* 11, 327–339.

COX CF, BERGENHOLTZ G, HEYS DR, SYED SA, FITZGERALD M, HEYS RJ (1985) Pulp capping of the dental pulp mechanically exposed to the oral microflora: a 1–2 year observation of wound healing in the monkey. *Journal of Oral Pathology* 14, 156–168.

PITT FORD TR, TORABINEJAD M, ABEDI H, BAKLAND LK, KARIAWASAM SP (1996) Using Mineral Trioxide Aggregate as a pulp-capping material. *Journal of the American Dental Association* 127, 1491–1494

SMITH AJ, MURRAY PE, LUMLEY PJ (2002) Preserving the vital pulp in operative dentistry: 1. A biological approach. *Dental Update* 29, 64–69.

SWIFT EJ, TROPE M, RITTER AV (2003) Vital pulp therapy for the mature tooth – can it work? *Endodontic Topics* 5, 49–56.

TORABINEJAD M, CHIVIAN N (1999) Clinical applications of Mineral Trioxide Aggregate. *Journal of Endodontics* 25, 197–205.

5 Root canal preparation

BYSTRÖM A, SUNDQVIST G (1981) Bacteriological evaluation of the efficacy of mechanical root canal instrumentation in endodontic therapy. *Scandinavian Journal of Dental Research* 89, 321–328.

BYSTRÖM A, SUNDQVIST G (1985) The antibacterial action of sodium hypochlorite and EDTA in 60 cases of endodontic therapy. *International Endodontic Journal* 18, 35–40.

DUMMER PM, MCGINN JH, REES DG (1984) The position and topography of the apical canal constriction and apical foramen. *International Endodontic Journal* 17, 192–198.

MARSHALL K (1990) RUBBER DAM. *British Dental Journal* 184, 218–219.

PITT FORD TR (2004) Pulp space anatomy and access cavities. In: Pitt Ford TR, ed. *Harty's Endodontics in Clinical Practice.* 5th edn. London, Wright.

PORTENIER I, WALTIMO TMT, HAAPASALO M (2003) *Enterococcus faecalis* – the root canal survivor and 'star' in post treatment disease. *Endodontic Topics* 6, 135–159.

SEN BH, WESSELINK PR (1995) The smear layer: a phenomenon in root canal therapy. *International Endodontic Journal* 28, 141–148.

SHUPING GB, ØRSTAVIK D, SIGURDSSON A, TROPE M (2000) Reduction of intracanal bacteria using nickel-titanium rotary instrumentation and various medicaments. *Journal of Endodontics* 26, 751–755.

SJÖGREN U, FIGDOR D, PERSSON S, SUNDQVIST G (1997) Influence of infection at the time of root filling on the outcome of endodontic treatment of teeth with apical periodontitis. *International Endodontic Journal* 30, 297–306.

SPANGBERG LS (1998) Endodontic treatment of teeth without apical periodontitis. In: Ørstavik D, Pitt Ford TR, (eds). *Essential Endodontology: prevention and treatment of apical periodontitis.* 1st edn. Oxford: Blackwell Science.

TORABINEJAD M, HANDYSIDES R, KHADEMI AA, BAKLAND LK (2002) Clinical implications of the smear layer in endodontics: a review. *Oral Surgery, Oral Medicine, Oral Pathology, Oral Radiology, Endodontics* 94, 658–666.

TROPE M (1990) Relationship of intracanal medicaments to endodontic flare-ups. *Endodontics and Dental Traumatology* 6, 226–229.

TROPE M, BERGENHOLTZ G (2002) Microbiological basis for endodontic treatment: can a maximal outcome be achieved in one visit? *Endodontic Topics* 1, 40–53.

6 Obturation of root canals

GUTMANN JL, WITHERSPOON DE (2002) Obturation of the cleaned and shaped root canal system. In: Cohen S, Burns RC (eds) *Pathways of the Pulp.* 8th edn. St Louis: Mosby.

HOMMEZ GMG, COPPENS CRM, DE MOOR RJG (2002). Periapical health related to the quality of coronal restorations and root fillings. *International Endodontic Journal* 35, 680–689.

LUSSI A, SUTER B, FRITZSCHE A, GYGAX M, PORTMANN P (2002) *In vivo* performance of the new non-instrumentation technology (NIT) for root canal obturation. *International Endodontic Journal* 35, 352–358.

SAUNDERS WP, SAUNDERS EM (1994) Coronal leakage as a cause of failure in root canal therapy: a review. *Endodontics and Dental Traumatology* 10, 105–108

7 Treatment outcomes

FRIEDMAN S (1998) Treatment outcome and prognosis of endodontic therapy. In: Ørstavik D, Pitt Ford TR, (eds). *Essential Endodontology: prevention and treatment of apical periodontitis.* 1st edn. Oxford: Blackwell Science.

RUBINSTEIN RA, KIM S (1999) Short-term observation of the results of endodontic surgery with the use of a surgical operating microscope and Super-EBA as root-end filling material. *Journal of Endodontics* 25, 43–48.

SUNDQVIST G, FIGDOR D, PERSSON S, SJÖGREN U (1998). Microbiological analysis of teeth with failed endodontic treatment and the outcome of conservative re-treatment. *Oral Surgery, Oral Medicine, Oral Pathology, Oral Radiology and Endodontics* 85, 86–93.

SIQUERIA JF (2001) Aetiology of root canal failure: why well-treated teeth can fail. *International Endodontic Journal* 34, 1–10.

8 Dealing with failure

BERGENHOLTZ G, SPÅNGBERG L (2004) Controversies in endodontics. *Critical Reviews in Oral Biology and Medicine* 15, 99–114.

GORNI FGM, GAGLIANI MM (2004) The outcome of endodontic retreatment: a 2-yr follow up. *Journal of Endodontics* 30, 1–4.

PITT FORD TR, MITCHELL PJC (2004) Problems in endodontic treatment. In: Pitt Ford TR, ed. *Harty's Endodontics in Clinical Practice.* **5th edn**. London, Wright.

RUDDLE CJ (2002) Nonsurgical endodontic retreatment. In: Cohen S, Burns RC (eds) *Pathways of the Pulp.* **8**th **edn**. St Louis: Mosby.

Section C

Self-assessment

Self-assessment

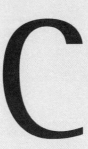

Self-assessment

Now is the time to ask yourself a few case-based questions. You might like to try these on your own or with a group of colleagues—you could arrange a quiz between groups. Whichever approach you adopt, please try to answer a few questions before dashing off to check the suggested answers (which are provided on page 187 onwards) as this will reduce artificiality. You will see that several questions assume you are working in general practice. The questions are arranged according to chapters of the preceding text.

A1 Introduction

(A) Standards of oral and dental health have a bearing upon the systemic health of our patients. What evidence is there to support this assertion and how might standards of endodontic care also influence the general health of patients?

(B) Make a list of all the possible advantages and disadvantages of the use of rubber dam in endodontic treatment. Arrange the lists in order of importance and identify the benefits to patient, operator, and treatment outcomes.

A2 The life of a tooth

(A) Try to imagine that you are a group of microorganisms intent on breaching the defences of a tooth. What are the obstacles that you are likely to encounter as you approach the pulp space and what conditions will improve your prospects of survival?

(B) Examine the section of pulp and dentine (which were shown in Fig. A2.9). Try to label as many structures as possible.

(C) List, in order of occurrence, lesions of non-endodontic origin that may be confused with periradicular disease induced by microorganisms.

A3 Diagnosis and treatment planning

(A)

(i) A male patient presents for a routine check up and remarks that he has had a recurrent 'gumboil on the side of his tooth'. Clinical examination reveals that there is a sinus adjacent to the lower right first molar tooth. After completing a history and intraoral examination, what are the special investigation(s) you would perform and what diagnosis is suspected?

(ii) How else may a sinus present?

(B) You investigate a multi-rooted tooth that, previously, has shown radiographic signs of periradicular pathology. However, vitality testing with an electric pulp tester gives a positive result, suggesting that the tooth is vital. What are the possible reasons for this apparently erroneous result?

(C)

(i) A patient presents complaining of a mobile anterior tooth. What are the possible causes?

(ii) What questions would you ask the patient?

(D) You make a diagnosis of irreversible pulpitis on a lower right first molar tooth. The dental history is vague but it is clear there is severe pain, preventing sleep. The medical history as reported shows the patient *may* suffer from hypertension. The dentition is heavily but well restored. There is no other pathology to be seen or elicited. The patient is elderly and lives in a residential home. They have made the trip to see you at the end of your working day with their daughter. The patient seems bemused but is far from uncooperative, yet their relative is putting pressure on you to 'get on with it and do something definitively and quickly', as her life is very busy. What would you do? Explain your reasons.

(E) In a case where there are multiple dental treatment needs, varying from extractions to simple oral hygiene therapy, at what point would you consider root canal treatment appropriate?

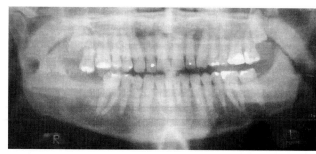

Fig. C3.1 Panoramic film showing unopposed UR 7.

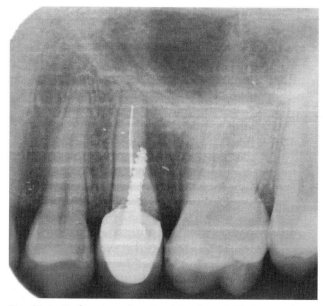

Fig. C3.2 Perforation of post-retained, root-filled premolar.

(F) A fit, healthy, highly motivated, 58-year-old male patient presents complaining of recurrent throbbing pain from his unopposed upper right second molar tooth (Fig. C3.1). A diagnosis of chronic periapical periodontitis is reached after clinical and radiographic examination. What are the treatment options you would discuss with the patient?

(G) A diagnosis of failing root canal treatment due to perforation is made on a fit and healthy 30-year-old patient (Fig. C3.2). What are the treatment options you would discuss with the patient?

A4 Preserving pulp vitality

(A)

(i) You are replacing an amalgam restoration because of signs of secondary caries. You have removed the entire restoration and upon final excavation of the dentine you expose the pulp iatrogenically. What should have been assessed prior to treating this patient?

(ii) How would you manage this case?

(iii) What would you advise the patient?

(B) Assume you are working in general practice. In conversation with colleagues you discover that they always treat both indirect and direct pulp exposures with Ledermix cement and a permanent restoration. They advise you that 'the treatment always works as patients never come back in pain—even when they presented with symptoms of lingering pain in the first place.' What do you think of this approach to treatment?

A5 Root canal preparation

(A)

(i) Whilst irrigating with sodium hypochlorite during root canal preparation of a maxillary molar tooth, the patient develops acute pain and swelling over the maxilla. The root canal is haemorrhaging heavily. What do you think has happened?

(ii) What is the immediate and long-term management of this patient?

(iii) How would you prevent this from occurring again?

(B)

(i) You have accessed and identified all the canal orifices in a previously untreated mandibular molar tooth. Canal patency is confirmed in the mesio-lingual canal, however you are unable to gain access to the full length of the mesio-buccal canal—it appears to be blocked apically. Why do you think this may be so?

(ii) What would be your next step?

(C) Your apex locator is giving inconsistent and erratic readings. What could be the possible reasons for this?

(D)

(i) During the later stages of root canal preparation a loss of working length is noted (a '0' apex locator reading was confirmed to be correct radiographically at the beginning of root treatment). What are the possible reasons for this loss of working length?

(ii) How may the probability of blocking the root canal be reduced?

A6 Obturation of root canals

(A) You have carried out root canal treatment on a tooth over two visits. At the end of the second visit your radiograph shows a root filling that is 2 mm shorter than the working length you expected it to reproduce. What are the possible causes and how can you avoid them?

(B) Why might there be voids in the root filling? Does it matter where these voids are?

(C) Your final radiograph shows a root filling that has extruded into the periapical tissues. Can you tell what (GP or sealer) has extruded and why? What is the significance of extrusion?

(D) A patient has had root canal preparation. He asks you how long can he leave the tooth in a temporized state before coming back for further treatment. What is your answer and why? He then tells you he does voluntary work in the third world and will not have access to a dentist for the next 3 months. What is your answer now? If this has changed, explain why.

(E) What is the role of apex locators in the obturation stage?

A7 Treatment outcomes

(A)

At a 1-year review of a completed root canal treatment the patient reports no symptoms. Clinically, the temporary dressing you placed has still not been replaced with a permanent restoration and radiographically there appears to be a radiolucent lesion. However, it has reduced significantly in size when compared with the pre-operative state. From the information given, answer the questions below.

(i) How would you categorize the outcome of this root canal treatment?

(ii) Would you review this case again? If you answer 'yes', when?

(iii) What advice would you give the patient?

(B) A patient presents 2 years after root canal treatment carried out by your predecessor. He is complaining of intermittent spontaneous episodes of discomfort and mild tenderness to biting localized to the root treated LR6 (Fig. C7.1). From the information given, answer the questions below.

(i) What is the outcome of the treatment?

(ii) What factors do you think have influenced the prognosis?

(iii) How would you explain your clinical findings to the patient and what are future treatment options?

A8 Dealing with failure

(A)

(i) Examine the pre-operative radiograph of a large maxillary lesion involving the maxilla (Fig. C8.1). All the teeth responded normally to thermal and electrical vitality tests. The lesion required surgical excision. Now look at a follow-up post-treatment radiograph (Fig. C8.2). Treatment appears successful. However, a number of teeth have received endodontic treatment, some with surgery. Can you offer an explanation for this?

(ii) Why, following treatment, do we find that five of the maxillary teeth have received endodontic treatment?

(B) The periradicular lesion related to the maxillary first premolar (Fig. C8.3) is of long standing. The tooth has recently become slightly tender to biting pressure. Can you suggest what the nature of the lesion is? Why is it persistent and why has the lesion not resolved following endodontic treatment? How would you manage this failure?

(C) A colleague has asked you to look at a patient for whom he has been trying to perform root canal treatment. The tooth in question is a central incisor (Fig. C8.4).

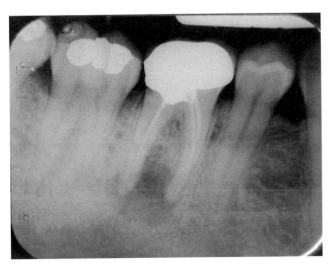

Fig. C7.1 The lower first molar was root treated 2 years ago and is symptomatic.

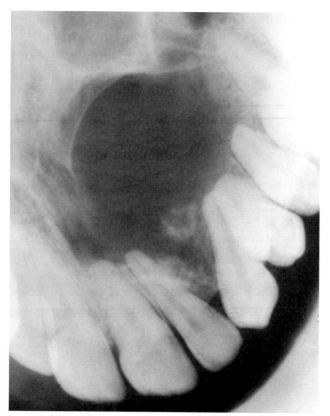

Fig. C8.1 A maxillary occlusal radiograph demonstrating a large, well-defined lesion. Note displacement of the lateral incisor and canine.

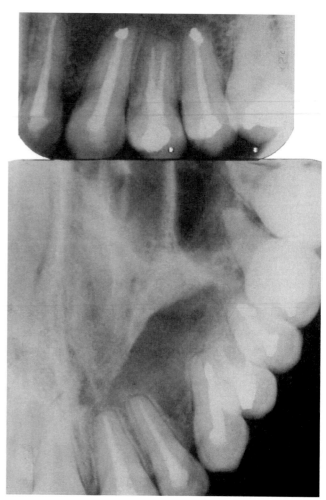

Fig. C8.2 Periapical and occlusal post-treatment radiographs of the case presented in Fig. C8.1. Endodontic treatment of five maxillary teeth, two of which have retrograde fillings is evident.

The patient originally reported with facial swelling, which subsided following the institution of drainage through the tooth. Since that time the canal has been instrumented on several occasions but the patient always returns complaining of tenderness in the tooth. Why is the tooth still tender? What would you advise should be done to settle the tooth? How would you manage the completion of the endodontic treatment?

(D) You have commenced root canal treatment for a mandibular first molar in one of your patients. During the negotiation of the very curved mesiobuccal canal a size 15, 0.02 taper, K-File fractures and the separated portion of the instrument is lodged in the middle third of the root canal. How would you explain the situation to your patient? Compose a letter of referral to a specialist colleague to seek their support in the completion of the treatment.

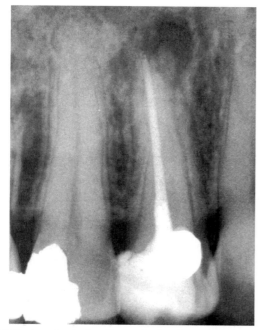

Fig. C8.3 A periapical radiograph of right maxillary premolars. The root-filled first premolar has a periapical radiolucency.

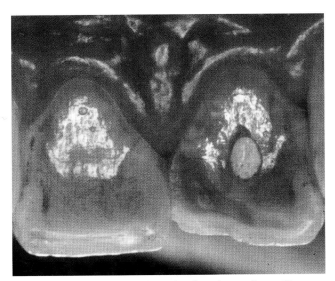

Fig. C8.4 Photograph of the palatal surfaces of maxillary central incisors. The fractured left central incisor is discoloured and there is an access cavity and provisional restoration.

Answers

A1 Introduction

(A) This question raises the long discussed issue that foci of infection within the oral tissues may influence general health. Current research has suggested that there might be a relationship between dental health and cardio-vascular disease. Several case reports have also suggested that dental sources may be the cause of systemic illnesses.

Whilst it has been confirmed that endodontic treatment can produce transient bacteraemias, there is no strong evidence to suggest that these foci of infection are the cause of systemic illnesses or infections.

There is not a simple 'yes' or 'no' to be provided and in order to answer this question fully you should review relevant literature and studies relating to the effects of dental health and endodontic treatment. You could try asking yourself questions about the potential impact upon patients with heart disease, rheumatoid arthritis, pyrexia of unknown origin and total hip replacement. The relevance of any bacteraemia must be appreciated when treating immunocompromised patients.

(B) The use of rubber dam as a barrier should be considered mandatory in the delivery of non-surgical root canal treatment. Failure to use rubber dam should be considered below acceptable clinical care.

The advantages for the use of rubber dam include:

- prevention of accidental loss of instruments into the respiratory or digestive tracts;
- improved infection control (reduction of saliva contamination);
- provision of a clean dry field of operation and improved visibility;
- giving a patient a sense of security and comfort;
- limiting (unhelpful) conversation;
- avoidance of a perceived need for frequent rinsing by the patient;
- avoidance of legal ramifications arising from non-use.

There are no disadvantages to using rubber dam, however, excuses such as it being:

- too difficult to use;
- time consuming;
- not tolerated by patients;

are claimed. None are substantiated. You should be in a position to comment on how each of the listed advantages is of benefit to the patient, operator or treatment outcome. The benefits of use far outweigh any perceived difficulties.

A2 The life af a tooth

(A) Each tooth is protected from the entry and action of microorganisms by a number of mechanisms, which include:

- the anti-bacterial properties of saliva;
- the physical integrity and impervious nature of enamel;
- the outward flow of dentinal tubular fluid;
- the formation of reparative dentine;
- the formation of peritubular dentine;
- the formation of reactionary dentine;
- intratubular calcifications;
- pulpal inflammatory reactions.

The potential for entry of microorganisms may be enhanced by conditions such as poor oral hygiene, dry mouth, fractured enamel, vascular damage to the pulp and loss of vitality of the tooth.

(B) The basic structural identification should include dentine, predentine, odontoblastic layer, cell-free and cell-rich sub-odontoblastic layers, and the pulp tissue proper. Within the pulp it is possible to identify blood vessels, fibroblasts and defence cells.

(C) Lesions of non-endodontic origin might include:

- periodontal lesions;

- idiopathic osteosclerosis;
- fibro-cemento-osseous dysplasia;
- other local and systemic pathology of non-endodontic origin.

A3 Diagnosis and treatment planning

(A)

(i) First, vitality test the tooth under suspicion as well as adjacent teeth. Second, track the origin of the sinus with a #20–25 GP point and expose a radiograph. These two investigations should confirm which tooth is associated with the sinus and it likely that the GP tip will be seen to be lying within an area of periradicular radiolucency. The diagnosis is likely to be one of chronic periradicular periodontitis with an associated sinus tract.

(ii) A sinus may discharge through the periodontal ligament, therefore 'walking' the probe around the tooth is essential to detect potentially narrow, deep, isolated probing depths.

(B) The patient may be very anxious and claim falsely to feel something to prevent further investigation (as they believe that the investigation will cause pain). Not all the roots may be necrotic in a multi-rooted tooth (therefore it is essential to test the buccal and palatal/lingual aspects of multi-rooted teeth). The metal electrode (if an electric pulp tester is being used) may be in contact with a metal restoration (amalgam/crown) or the gingivae. Liquefaction necrosis in a necrotic pulp may conduct the current to the adjacent periodontal ligament. Poor isolation of the tooth under investigation may result in saliva acting as an electrical conductor (if an electric pulp tester is being used).

(C)

(i)

- Loss of periodontal attachment—as a result of periodontal or endodontic disease;
- Excessive occlusal trauma/interferences;
- dento-alveolar trauma;
- decemented post-crown restoration;
- pathology.

(ii)

- Does the tooth in question hurt (if so what is the character of the pain)?
- How long has the tooth been mobile and is it getting worse?

- Has the increasing mobility occurred gradually or suddenly?
- Has there been any recent dental treatment?
- Has the tooth been traumatized in an accident (e.g. sports injury or a fight)?

(D) You must act in the best interests of the patient at all times. The options for irreversible pulpitis are clear: extraction or root canal treatment—these should be discussed with the patient and daughter. It would be sensible not to perform an extraction at this visit, as you cannot be sure of the medical history without confirmation from the patient's general practitioner or the patient's ability to give informed consent—ask for agreement that you will contact their GP. Root canal treatment may be the correct option. However, at this visit the pulp should only be extirpated and the tooth dressed with Ledermix® paste and a well adapted temporary restoration to help the patient out of pain. Review the patient when all relevant medical history information has been provided and you are able to ascertain (with the general practitioner's advice) if the patient is able to give informed consent.

(E) As in the previous example, it is essential to make a judgement in the best interests of each patient before committing them to time-consuming and possibly expensive treatment. In this case, it would be wise to stage the treatment plan such that after initial, simple and essential treatments (e.g. extraction of teeth with a hopeless prognosis, institution of a preventive regime, stabilization of frank caries with temporary dressings or simple plastic restorations) time is made available specifically for detailed re-assessment of patient motivation (for example, improved plaque control and attendance) before embarking on root canal treatment.

Looking at the case slightly more broadly, relatively straightforward root canal treatments may be indicated on anterior teeth during the initial phase but again, re-assessment would be needed before commencing such treatments on posterior teeth. Patient expectations of dental treatment tend to show differences depending on geographical location and within and between countries, and this should be taken into account. What is 'correct' in one situation is not in another.

(F)

- Root canal treatment (the tooth is unopposed and therefore is redundant): root treating the tooth to retain it would only be worthwhile if restoration of the opposing saddle with an implant was planned.

- Extraction (this option may be the most desirable as the tooth is not in function).

- Leave and monitor (the patient *must* be advised that he will most likely suffer from recurrent pain and/or swelling from this tooth and the notes should be documented accordingly)—not an ideal option.

(G)

- Re-root canal treatment—refer to a specialist Endodontist. The prognosis will be dependent on removing the post crown without fracturing the root and being able to seal the perforation.

- Extraction—the resulting gap may be restored with a single unit implant or a bridge if the patient is not happy with a gap.

- Leave and monitor—the patient *must* be aware of the problem and possible sequelae (you should discuss what these are) and the notes *must* be documented appropriately and contemporaneously to indicate that this is not an ideal option.

A4 Preserving pulp vitality

(A)

(i)

- Presence of any symptoms or signs that indicate the status of the pulp (i.e. healthy or reversibly inflamed versus irreversibly inflamed/necrotic pulp).

- Radiograph—the proximity of the carious lesion to the pulp and signs of periradicular involvement.

(ii) Place rubber dam (if already not in place). Perform pulp-capping procedure (assuming there were no symptoms or signs of irreversible damage).

(iii)

- Why a pulp preservation procedure was being performed instead of a 'normal' restoration (or root canal treatment). Obtain consent prior to carrying out the treatment.

- Importance of follow-up appointments as root canal treatment may be required in the future.

(B) The use of steroid-based medicaments is not a good idea in the long term as any inflamed condition of the pulp will be suppressed, therefore the pulp will die quietly and eventually become infected.

A5 Root canal preparation

(A)

(i) This situation is called a 'hypochlorite accident' and is caused by sodium hypochlorite inadvertently entering the periodontal tissues via the apical foramen.

(ii)

Immediate management

- Be calm and reassure the patient;

- Advise them of what has happened;

- Irrigate the canals with saline, then dry and temporize the canal and access cavity;

- Prescribe analgesics for pain relief and antibiotics;

- Advise the patient that swelling may take up to a week to reduce fully and that bruising is quite common but should subside again after a short period of time;

- Document the incident in the patient's records;

- Review patient in 2–3 days.

Longer term management

When the patient is stable, consider completing treatment.

(iii)

- Always pre-measure the irrigant syringe needle so that it is several mm short of the working length.

- Never force the needle as it should sit passively in the canal. Do not use excessive force on the syringe's plunger (this can be reduced by using a forefinger rather than a thumb on the plunger).

(B)

(i) The mesial canals join apically.

(ii) This should be confirmed by taking a radiograph with a file to the full working length in the mesio-lingual canal and another file to the point in the mesio-buccal canal where it stops abruptly.

If an apex locator is available, place a file to the '0' reading length in the mesio-lingual canal, then place another file in the mesio-buccal canal and attach the apex locator lead to it. When this file reaches the 'blockage' (it should be in contact with the file in the mesio-lingual canal and thus complete the electrical circuit), the apex locator readout will confirm a '0' reading again.

(C)

* Liquid (irrigant/pus/blood) in the pulp chamber;
* File contacting a metallic restoration;
* Vital tissue apically;
* Very large apical foramen;
* Low battery.

(D)

(i)

* The canal may be blocked with debris or aberrations created;
* If the canal was moderately to severely curved there may be a small (<1 mm) reduction in working length as the canal curvature always reduces slightly with preparation.

(ii)

* Use a crown-down preparation technique and do not skip file sizes;
* Copious irrigation between file sizes;
* Recapitulation with the largest file that goes to working length.

A6 Obturation of root canals

(A) It must be remembered that in almost all cases, the result of the obturation is due to the quality of preparation. The possible problems at the preparation stage that can result in a short root filling are as follows:

* Inadequacy of access and preparation of the root canals to the full working length due to:
  * poor understanding of the anatomy and not noticing root canals divide apically;
  * inability to follow root canal curvature during instrumentation;
* Blocking the apical portion of the root canal with:
  * debris (canal lack of irrigation, recapitulation, and maintaining due to patency);
  * a separated instrument;
  * poor preparation resulting in ledging of the root canal.
* The obturation stage may also result in short root filling through:
  * inappropriate master point selection (too large);
  * inappropriate placement of master GP point (buckling);

It must also be emphasized that any technical problem in relation to working length may be due to lack of reference point accuracy and incorrect use of apex locators.

(B) Voids generally occur due to poor obturation technique. If there has been an inadequate amount of GP and sealer used there will, inevitably, be voids.

Other reasons include poor preparation (shape and taper) of the root canal. Common causes of voids include:

* poor master cone selection (wrong size);
* accessory GP points buckling during placement;
* poor finger spreader placement (it needs to follow the outer (convex) side of the curve to allow for placement of the greatest number of points);
* poor accessory GP placement (insufficient number or not being placed where the finger spreader made space);
* insufficient pressure during compaction;
* inadequate amount of sealer;
* presence of ledges from the preparation stage not allowing GP and or finger spreader to follow the root canal shape.
* poor taper of the prepared canal.

Positions of voids are important. A small void in the mid-third (with master cone to the correct length) may not be as crucial as a large void in the coronal third, which may be very susceptible to microleakage. In general terms, assess voids and their risk potential for the recurrence of disease:

* size;
* position;
* patient factors (for example, co-operation for re-root canal treatment);
* quality of the future coronal seal.

(C) Two materials may extrude: GP and sealer. Gutta percha normally appears as a solid, radiopaque mass on a radiograph. If it is 'thick' in appearance it is probably the master GP point. Sealer extrusion appears more like a puff of cement and is much finer in size than GP extrusion.

Master GP points may extrude due to either or both of the following:

* lack of resistance of the root canal shape (over-instrumentation, poor apical preparation and step back, lack of taper)
* poor selection of master GP (too small a point).

Accessory points extrude due to:

♦ inadequate measurement of finger spreader and cones;

♦ too much pressure on the finger spreader;

♦ poor adaptation of the master GP point.

(D) The waiting period between preparation and obturation visits is generally assumed to be 1 week (minimum). The treatment should then be completed so that a permanent restoration can be placed on the tooth. If the patient has to leave the tooth for a few weeks before returning, this should not present a problem as long as the temporary restoration is of good quality. If he is unable to attend for a number of months then the temporary restoration should comprise a base of IRM with a layer of a stronger material over it (for example, glass ionomer). You may also want to advise for the patient to take a travel kit for teeth (which contains dressing materials) should the temporary restoration be lost.

(E) Apex locators can be used at this stage to:

♦ reconfirm zero reading and indirectly the working length;

♦ make sure canal patency has not been lost (that is, that the canals are not blocked, for example, with debris, calcium hydroxide, or previous root canal filling material);

♦ check for perforations or other iatrogenic injuries.

A7 Treatment outcomes

(A)

(i) The treatment may be regarded as a success endodontically as there has been a reduction in the size of the periapical radiolucency. This is despite the presence of a temporary restoration.

(ii) The tooth should be reviewed again in approximately 1 year.

(iii) Advise the patient that root treatment appears to be a success and that it would be desirable to re-assess the tooth again at their next check up appointment. Strongly advise the patient to have the tooth permanently restored – leaving the temporary restoration may have a negative influence on the prognosis.

(B)

(i) Failed root canal treatment.

(ii) The most likely cause of failure is persistent/residual infection due to the root canal system not being ade-

quately prepared and obturated. From the radiographs, the root filling (and therefore preparation) appears to be 5–6mm short of the desired working length.

There is also a possibility that additional canal(s) may not have been identified (40+% of mandibular first molars have 2 distal canals).

There also appear to be signs of a poor distal margin on the existing restoration (coronal leakage) that may also be a contributory factor.

(iii) Advise the patient that their symptoms appear to be most likely due to persistent infection within the root canals. Treatment options are: leave alone (not advised), re-root canal treatment or extraction.

A8 Dealing with failure

(A)

(i) The lesion is not of endodontic origin (for example, it may be a developmental cyst).

(ii) It is possible that, prior to the excision of the large lesion, a decision was made to undertake root canal treatment of the teeth closely associated with the lesion. Presumably the risk of vascular damage to the pulps of these teeth drove the decision. It also appears that, during the surgical excision of the lesion, two of the teeth received retrograde seals. An alternative approach to treatment might have involved decompression rather than excision. The endodontic treatment of the teeth could have been avoided by post-treatment monitoring of the vitality of the teeth associated with the lesion.

(B) The lesion related to the maxillary first premolar is chronic periradicular periodontitis. The tenderness is the result of inflammation induced by microorganisms and their products. This periradicular periodontitis is usually treated by the removal of the contents of the pulp space followed by disinfection and sealing. This lesion has not resolved because of the persistent effects of the microorganisms and their products. Management requires the identification of untreated pulp space using horizontal parallax techniques. In this case, failure to treat a second root canal should be suspected. Endodontic re-treatment should then be considered.

(C) Persistent tenderness indicates the presence of inflammation induced by microorganisms and their products. The primary objective of treatment should be the shaping and disinfection of the pulp space followed by adequate sealing to prevent re-infection. The photograph suggests that the palatal access is inadequate. It is also possible to identify one of the pulp horns in the incisal fracture. Management requires opening and improving the shape and size of the access cavity followed by the shaping, cleaning, and thorough disinfection of the pulp space. The placement of an intracanal medicament (for example, calcium hydroxide) would further assist in the disinfection process prior to the completion of the root canal treatment.

(D) Anyone who performs endodontic treatment on a regular basis will experience at some stage the fracture of an instrument. Whenever this type of incident occurs the patient should be informed immediately and the position separated instrument located radiographically. An assessment of the effect that the incident has upon continuing treatment should also be given. In the case of a fractured instrument in the middle third of the root canal it is often possible to remove or bypass the blockage and continue the treatment. Where specialist advice and treatment is sought, a comprehensive letter should be forwarded to the specialist giving the following details:

◆ full patient details including medical history;

◆ history of the present problem;

◆ radiographs;

◆ an outline of the restorative treatment plan.

Index